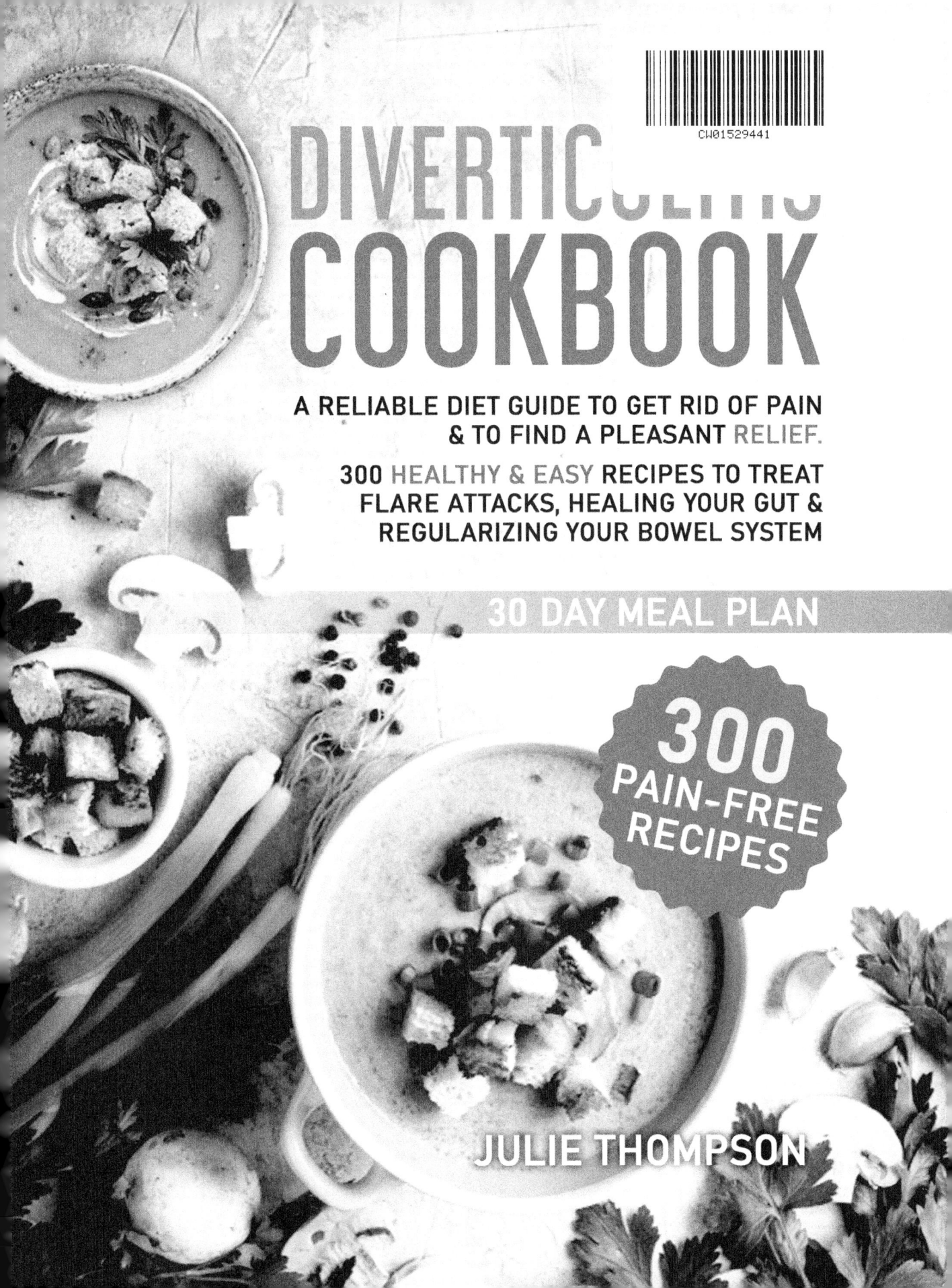

Julie Thompson © Copyright 2021

All rights reserved.

This document's objective is to provide accurate and dependable information about the subject and issue at hand. The publisher sells the book with the knowledge that it is not bound to provide accounting, legally permissible, or otherwise qualifying services. If legal or professional assistance is required, it is prudent to consult a knowledgeable specialist.

From a Declaration of Principles that an American Bar Association Committee and a Publishers and Associations Committee jointly recognized and approved.

No portion of this publication, whether electronic or printed, may be reproduced, duplicated, or transmitted in any form or by any means. It is highly illegal to record this publication, and storage of this document is permitted only with the publisher's prior consent.

The material presented below is declared to be accurate and consistent, with the caveat that any liability resulting from the use or abuse of any policies, processes, or directions contained herein, whether due to inattention or otherwise, is entirely the recipient reader's duty. The publisher shall not be accountable for any compensation, damages, or monetary loss experienced as a result of the information included herein, whether directly or indirectly.

The writers retain all copyrights not held by the publisher.

The information presented on this page is primarily educational in nature and is hence universal. The information is provided "as is" with no implied commitment or guarantee.

The trademarks are utilized without the permission or backing of the trademark owner, and the trademark is published without the consent or backing of the trademark owner. All trademarks and registered trademarks referenced in this book are the property of their respective owners and are not associated with this publication.

TABLE OF CONTENTS

INTRODUCTION	5
CHAPTER 1: WHAT IS DIVERTICULITIS?	7
CHAPTER 2: HOW TO TREAT DIVERTICULITIS	12
CHAPTER 3: HOW TO PREVENT DIVERTICULITIS FLARE-UPS WITH FOOD	26
CHAPTER 4: YES FOODS VS NO FOODS FOR EACH PHASE OF DIVERTICULITIS	32
CHAPTER 5: BREAKFAST (CLEAR FLUIDS)	39
CHAPTER 6: LUNCH (CLEAR FLUIDS)	72
CHAPTER 7: DINNER (CLEAR FLUIDS)	106
CHAPTER 8: SNACKS (CLEAR FLUIDS)	113
CHAPTER 9: BREAKFAST (LOW-RESIDUE)	126
CHAPTER 10: LUNCH (LOW-RESIDUE)	136
CHAPTER 11: DINNER (LOW-RESIDUE)	143
CHAPTER 12: BREAKFAST (FIBER-RICH)	147
CHAPTER 13: LUNCH (FIBER-RICH)	152
CHAPTER 14: SNACKS (FIBER-RICH)	172
YOUR 30-DAY MEAL PLAN	181
CONCLUSION	186
RECIPE INDEX	188

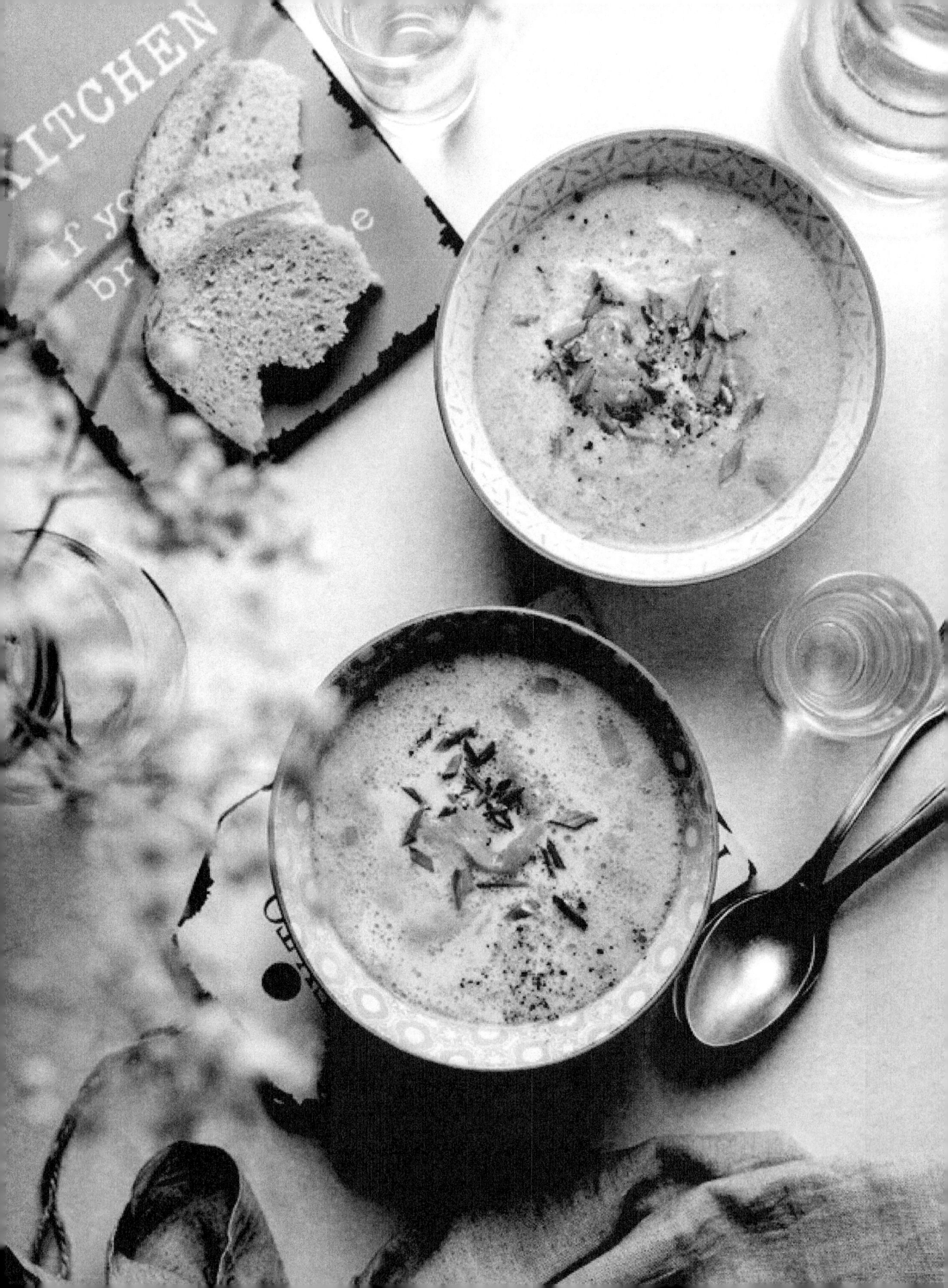

INTRODUCTION

Diverticulitis is caused by a condition known as diverticulosis. People over the age of 40 are more likely to have this disease. Diverticula affect more than half of all individuals over the age of 60 in the United States. Diverticula may develop everywhere in the body, including the esophagus, stomach, and small intestine, although they seem to occur more often in the large intestine.

Diverticular issues are known to be caused by a low-fiber diet. The emergence of diverticular illness coincided with low-fiber processed foods such as brainless refined flour in the early 1900s, and it is now prevalent across many developed nations. And, in places like Asia and Africa, this illness is uncommon because people consume a lot of high-fiber foods.

Diverticulitis is similar to appendicitis in that it causes pain in the lower left side of the abdomen, which is where most individuals in the West are afflicted. Although appendicitis pain is most often felt on the lower right side, diverticulitis pain is usually severe and comes abruptly. You may initially feel minor pain that grows worse after a few days and varies in severity.

Abdominal pain, fever, nausea, and constipation or diarrhea are among the additional symptoms. Then there are the less common indications and symptoms, including nausea, bloating, rectum hemorrhage, repeated urination, discomfort when peeing, and abdominal soreness while wearing a belt or bending over. To identify symptoms of diverticulitis, doctors will utilize x-rays taken after a barium or gastrogaffin enema, a sigmoidoscopy, or a colonoscopy.

Many physicians advise patients with diverticulosis to avoid seeds and nuts, including tiny seeds found in foods like tomatoes and strawberries. These tiny particles were thought to become stuck in the diverticula and induce irritation. There is, however, no scientific evidence to support this idea. In fact, eating a high-fiber diet rich in nuts and seeds lowers the incidence of diverticulitis. People are now more inclined to believe that only foods that irritate or get stuck in the diverticula cause difficulties.

During any flare-up phases of diverticulitis, a low residue Diverticulitis Diet is suggested to decrease stool volume and heal the affected region. A low residue Diverticulitis Diet has fewer than 10 grams of fiber per day. If you've been on this diet for a long period, your doctor may recommend that you take daily multivitamin-mineral tablets.

The therapy will usually be determined by the severity of the symptoms, including the presence of diverticulitis. If your symptoms are minor, antibiotics plus a liquid or low-fiber diet can suffice. However, if you're at risk of additional problems or have repeated episodes of diverticulitis, you may need more sophisticated treatment. A high-fiber diet is necessary to avoid recurrent diverticulitis outbreaks. In addition, when you increase your fiber consumption, you should also increase your hydration intake.

The diverticulitis diet is used to treat patients who have diverticulitis, which typically affects people over the age of 60, although it may also affect persons as young as 20.

A diverticulitis diet consists of a low residue diet that promotes a decrease in bowel movement in order to reduce the infection and improve healing of the inflamed diverticula in the early stages of the disease.

The low fiber diverticulitis diet consists of eating fewer than 10 grams of fiber per day. A low-fiber diverticulitis diet necessitates the use of regular mineral and vitamin supplements.

As a person's symptoms improve, they may begin a high-fiber diverticulitis diet by increasing their daily fiber consumption from 5 to 15 grams. This will give the digestive system time to adapt to the increased fiber in their diet.

Constipation should be avoided at all costs since it may worsen a person's illness. The fundamental concept of a high fiber diverticulitis diet is to increase daily fiber consumption while also maintaining a high hydration intake.

The high fiber diverticulitis diet is intended to aid digestive system healing during the acute stage of diverticulitis. In contrast, the low fiber diverticulitis diet is intended to prevent recurrent diverticulitis attacks.

Most people are unaware of the dangers of a low-fiber diet, and the Diverticulitis Diet may help anybody. To provide the body with necessary nutrients, we must incorporate high-fiber foods into our diets. Even if you have diverticulitis, the Diverticulitis Dieting plan will undoubtedly assist you in regaining control of your body's nutrition and achieving a good and healthy body state.

You can start by looking up different types of high-fiber diets for Diverticulitis online; for example, Google "Diverticulitis Diet Plans," and you should find dozens of sites with the information you need; however, I would recommend that you only pay attention to this reputable book because you don't want to waste time on bogus information that will do you no good.

CHAPTER 1: WHAT IS DIVERTICULITIS?

According to the National Institutes of Health, diverticulosis is a disease in which diverticula are present in the gut. Still, there are no symptoms of inflammation or bleeding, and it does not produce diverticulitis or diverticular bleeding.

Diverticulosis is often discovered during regular X-rays or colonoscopies. Constipation, diarrhea, persistent cramping or discomfort in the lower abdomen, and bloating are common symptoms; however, some individuals suffer constipation, diarrhea, chronic cramping or pain in the lower abdomen, and bloating. According to the National Institutes of Health, people who are experiencing these symptoms should get medical assistance from their health care practitioner, since other diseases such as irritable bowel syndrome and stomach ulcers may produce similar issues.

Diverticulosis may be treated with a high-fiber diet, fiber supplements, medicines, or even probiotics in certain cases.

Diverticular Illness occurred when tiny sacs or pouches called diverticulum develop and push outward via weak areas in the colon wall, causing diverticular disease. Diverticula are a collection of pouches.

People above the age of 50 are more likely to develop diverticulosis. Diverticulitis develops in certain individuals who have diverticulosis. Diverticular illness has been growing more prevalent in individuals under the age of 50 in recent years.

While the precise etiology of diverticulosis and diverticular disease is unknown, it is thought that both are caused by a low-fiber diet.

Diverticulosis and diverticular disease were first observed in the United States in the early 1900s and are thought to have been caused by a diet high in processed foods with little fiber. Both diseases are especially prevalent in the United States, England, and Australia, all of which have low-fiber diets.

According to other studies, low serotonin levels induced reduced relaxation and increased colon muscular spasms, which may lead to diverticulosis and diverticular disease. Obesity, lack of exercise, smoking, and certain medicines have all been linked to diverticular illness.

Symptoms

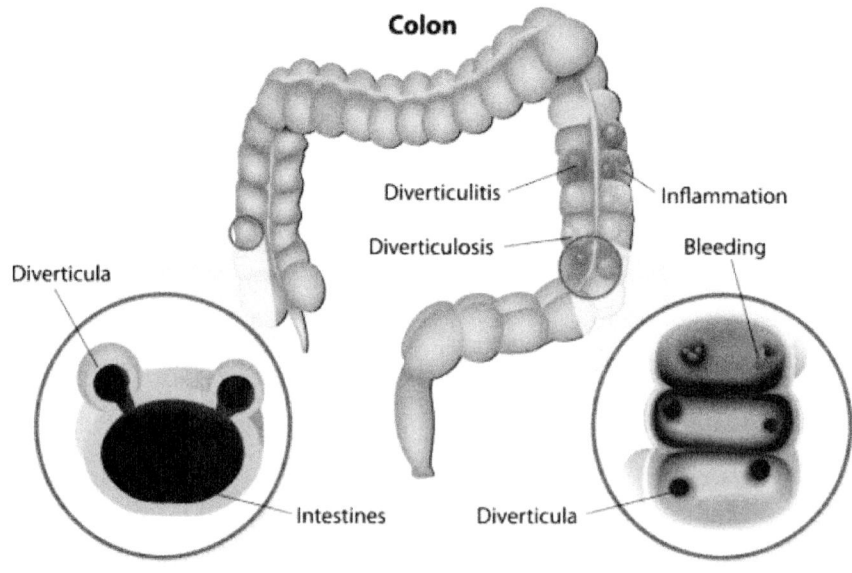

Diverticulosis and diverticulitis have distinct symptoms.

Diverticulosis symptoms

The majority of people with diverticulosis have no symptoms at all. Asymptomatic diverticulosis is the term for this condition.

There may be discomfort in the lower abdomen at times. More particularly, the lower-left portion of the abdomen is typically affected. The discomfort usually occurs when the person eats or passes feces. After breaking wind, there may be some relief.

Other symptoms include:

- » Constipation and, less commonly, diarrhea
- » Changing bowel habits
- » Small amounts of blood in stools

Diverticulitis symptoms

When diverticulitis becomes inflamed, symptoms include:

- » Painful urination
- » Fever

- » Constant and usually severe pain, usually on the left side of the abdomen although occasionally on the right
- » More frequent urination
- » Nausea and vomiting
- » Bleeding from the rectum

When to see a doctor

If you experience persistent, unexplained stomach discomfort, get medical help right once, especially if you also have a fever, constipation, or diarrhea.

FACTORS THAT INCREASE CHANCES OF DEVELOPING DIVERTICULITIS

Diverticula develop when the colon's inherently weak regions break away under stress. As a consequence, marble-sized pockets develop through the colon wall.

A tear in the diverticula produces inflammation and, in rare cases, infection, resulting in diverticulitis.

Risk factors

Diverticulitis may result from a variety of factors, including:

- » Aging. Diverticulitis becomes more common as people become older.
- » Obesity. You're more likely to have diverticulitis if you're very overweight.
- » Smoking. People who smoke cigarettes are more prone to get diverticulitis than nonsmokers.
- » Lack of physical activity. Diverticulitis seems to be reduced by vigorous exercise.
- » It is suggested that you eat a diet high in animal fat and low in fiber. Although the effect of low fiber alone is unclear, a low-fiber diet in conjunction with high consumption of animal fat seems to raise the risk.
- » Medications in particular. Several medications, including steroids, opioids, and nonsteroidal anti-inflammatory drugs like ibuprofen (Advil, Motrin IB, and others), have been linked to an increased risk of diverticulitis (Aleve).

Complications

About 25% of people with acute diverticulitis develop complications, which may include:

- » When pus accumulates in the pouch, it becomes an abscess.

- » Scarring obstructs your intestines.

- » A fistula is an irregular channel between parts of the intestine or between the colon and other organs.

- » Peritonitis is a condition that occurs when an infected or inflammatory pouch ruptures, allowing intestinal contents to flow into the abdominal cavity. Peritonitis is a medical emergency that requires urgent medical attention.

Prevention

To help prevent diverticulitis:

- » Exercise on a regular basis. Exercise helps to maintain regular bowel function and lowers colon pressure. On most days, try to exercise for at least 30 minutes.

- » Increase your fiber intake. Diverticulitis is less likely if you eat a high-fiber diet. Fresh fruits and vegetables and whole grains are high in fiber, which softens waste and allows it to move through your colon more rapidly. Diverticulitis is not linked to the consumption of seeds and nuts.

- » Drink a lot of water. Fiber absorbs water and increases the amount of soft, bulky waste in your colon. On the other hand, fiber may cause constipation if you don't drink enough fluids to replenish what's been absorbed.

- » Smoking should be avoided. Smoking has been linked to a higher incidence of diverticulitis.

WHEN IS DIVERTICULOSIS DANGEROUS

Diverticulitis is a potentially fatal disease in which pockets of diverticula develop in the colon and become inflamed. These pockets may cause severe abdominal discomfort and can lead to death if not treated correctly and quickly. While this disease is often managed with medicine and a change in diet, there are certain signs to watch for that indicate when you should go to the emergency department for diverticulitis.

Diverticulitis has a few symptoms that should never be overlooked. These symptoms indicate a more serious development of the disease, which usually necessitates a two-day hospital stay for IV antibiotics and surgery in more severe instances. Symptoms include excessive vomiting and severe nausea, a fever of above 100°F with or without chills, and a loss or sudden change in appetite.

Because the emergency room may be a frightening environment, an increasing number of patients are discovering that stand-alone emergency departments are a better match for their requirements. Physicians Premier, for example, provides the same services like hospitals, but without the hospital setting. If treatment necessitates a hospital stay, the facility will provide transportation to the hospital. In any event, if you have any of the severe symptoms of diverticulitis, or if you have symptoms that may be a sign of anything more serious, you should get treatment as soon as possible.

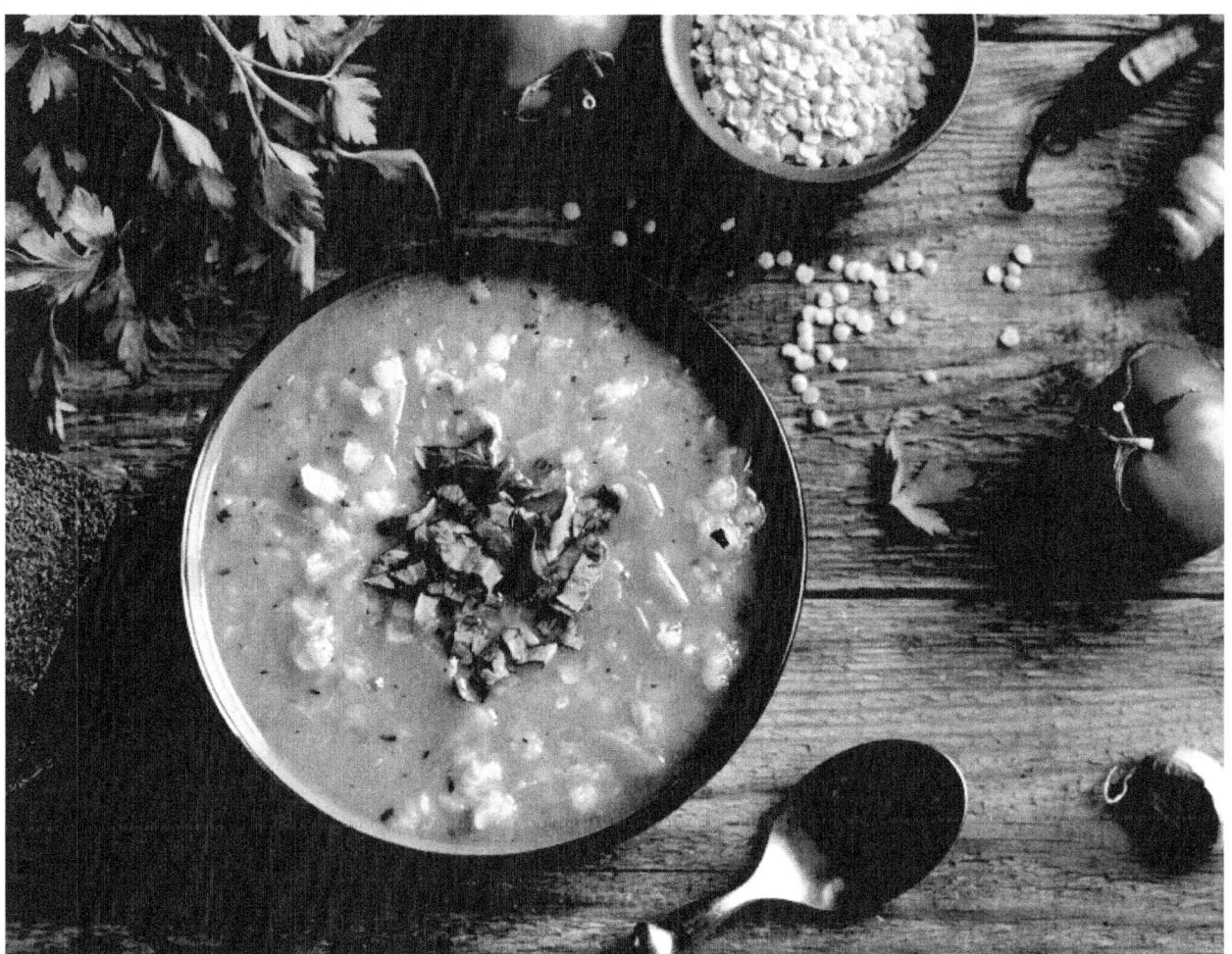

CHAPTER 2: HOW TO TREAT DIVERTICULITIS

Unless you have your diverticula surgically removed, which is not typically done, you will have them for the rest of your life. By altering your diet, you may reduce your chances of contracting an illness. Suppose you have a moderate case of diverticulosis. In that case, your doctor may recommend that you consume a high-fiber diet to keep your bowels moving and decrease your chances of developing diverticulitis.

If you get diverticulitis, you should consult a doctor to ensure a full recovery and prevent potentially fatal consequences. Diverticulitis is treated with diet changes, antibiotics, and potentially surgery.

Bed rest, stool softeners, a liquid diet, antibiotics to combat the infection, and potentially antispasmodic medications may be used to treat mild diverticulitis infection.

If you have a perforation or a more serious infection, you will most likely be admitted to the hospital and given antibiotics intravenously (via a vein). You may also be fed intravenously to allow your intestines to heal. In addition, your doctor may recommend a temporary colostomy to drain infected abscesses and relax the digestive system. Your intestine will drain into a bag connected to the front of your belly after a colostomy produces an opening (called a stoma). This technique may be reversed during a second surgery, depending on the outcome of the recovery.

If you've had multiple episodes of acute diverticulitis, your doctor may recommend that you have the damaged portion of your intestine removed after you're no longer experiencing symptoms. If intravenous treatment fails to treat an acute episode of diverticulitis successfully, surgery may be required. Whatever therapy you get, your chances of making a complete recovery are extremely high if you seek medical help as soon as possible.

To avoid constipation, drink at least eight 8-ounce glasses of water each day. Prunes or prune juice may be used as a natural laxative if you get constipated. Low-fat diets are recommended because fat inhibits the transit of food through the gut.

While the diverticula are inflamed and sensitive during an acute episode of diverticulitis, stick to clear liquids or broths.

Cooked vegetables, cooked fruits, and apples are rich in fiber and may be beneficial during times of remission. Probiotics, which may be found in yogurt, may also be beneficial.

Your doctor may recommend the following to treat complications of diverticulitis:

Abscess

If an abscess is big or does not respond to medication, your doctor may recommend draining it.

Perforation

A perforation will almost certainly require surgery to fix the rip or hole. If the surgeon is unable to heal the perforation, further surgery to remove a small portion of your colon may be required.

Peritonitis

Peritonitis needs urgent surgery to clear out your abdomen. After a course of antibiotics, you may require a colon resection at a later date. If you've lost a lot of blood, you may require a blood transfusion. Peritonitis may be deadly if not treated quickly.

Fistula

A fistula may be repaired by a surgeon conducting a colon resection and eliminating the fistula.

Intestinal obstruction

You will require immediate surgery with potential colon resection if your big intestine is obstructed. Because partial blockage is not an emergency, surgery or other remedial treatments may be scheduled.

4 Stages According To Hinchey Classification Of Acute Diverticuliti

The Hinchey Classification is used to classify colon perforations caused by diverticulitis. Dr. E John Hinchey (1934–present), a general surgeon at the Montreal General Hospital and a professor of surgery at McGill University, created the categorization.

Diverticulosis, or the presence of intestinal diverticula, is a very common occurrence. As individuals become older, pressure from the interior of the intestine pulls the mucosa outwardly, causing out-pouching of the intestinal wall. The pouches (diverticula) form when there is a gap between or weakening within the gut wall's muscle fibers, most often at locations of vascular protrusion into the wall. Although the majority of diverticula are asymptomatic, the bloody stool is the most frequent sign of diverticula. Diverticulitis is a disease that develops when the diverticula (singular: diverticulum) gets inflamed and becomes an inflammation site. Lower abdomen discomfort, changes in bowel habits (diarrhea or constipation), and indications of inflammation (fever/chills, nausea/vomiting) are all common symptoms. Diverticulitis, unlike diverticulosis (the condition of having outpouchings), is seldom accompanied by active bleeding.

Diverticulitis may cause a number of problems, including perforation of the intestine, which is one of the most severe ones. In this context, "perforation" refers to the rupture of the diverticulum, which causes air to flow into the abdominal cavity. It is possible to conceal a hole if it is extremely tiny (often referred to by surgeons as a localized perforation). If it is not confined, it may cause fecal peritonitis (fecal infection of the peritoneal cavity), which is frequently deadly.

STAGES OF DIVERTICULITIS

According to the Hinchey classification, there are four phases of diverticulitis:

Stage 1: Diverticulitis accompanied by phlegmon or a mesenteric or pericolic abscess. This indicates the presence of inflammatory masses or abscesses in the fat surrounding the colon or the small intestine folds.

Stage 2: Diverticulitis accompanied by phlegmon or a mesenteric or pericolic abscess. This indicates the presence of inflammatory masses or abscesses in the fat surrounding the colon or the small intestine folds.

Stage 3: Generalized purulent peritonitis due to perforated diverticulitis. This indicates that the abscesses have ruptured and the inflammation is causing pus to leak into the belly.

Stage 4: Diverticula rupture into the peritoneal cavity, resulting in fecal contamination and widespread fecal peritonitis. This indicates that the abscesses have burst into the peritoneal cavity, producing an infection due to feces in the peritoneal cavity due to the rupture.

"If the diverticula are burst, the patient may need surgical removal of part of the sigmoid colon, but minor instances are typically managed with a clear liquid diet and antibiotics," says Dr. Francisco Itriago MD. FOR EXAMPLE, Stages III and IV diverticulitis have burst abscesses that would almost certainly need surgery, while Stages I and II do not.

How To Behave For Every One Of Them

Around half of all Americans have or have had diverticulosis by the age of 60. Women are more likely than males to get diverticulitis beyond the age of 50, while men are more likely to develop it before the age of 50. Diverticulosis affects almost everyone over the age of 80, although not everyone with diverticulitis.

Diverticulitis is responsible for about 3,000 fatalities each year in the United States, with an estimated 2 million individuals suffering from the condition.

The treatment of individuals with diverticulitis is determined by the severity of their symptoms, the existence of complications, and any concomitant diseases. As a result, there is no standard therapy for diverticular illness, including diverticulitis, in medical practice.

The first step is to figure out if the patient has a complex or simple illness. Uncomplicated diverticulitis is described as localized diverticular inflammation without complication. In contrast, complicated diverticulitis is defined as inflammation that is accompanied by a complication such as an abscess, a fistula, blockage, bleeding, or perforation. CT imaging can confirm the diagnosis of diverticulitis and differentiate between the two disease stages.

Uncomplicated diverticulitis may be treated medically and in an outpatient environment. At the same time, complicated illness requires a more aggressive approach, which may include urgent or elective surgery, as well as therapies tailored to the problem (e.g., abscess drainage). A gastrointestinal consultation, as well as surgical and interventional radiology consults, may be beneficial. The modified Hinchey classification, based on CT scan results, is used to classify diverticulitis and suggest suitable treatments.

An emergency colectomy is done when serious problems develop or the patient's condition does not respond to medical therapy. Purulent peritonitis, uncontrolled sepsis, fistula, and blockage are all complications that need surgical intervention. Approximately 20% of patients hospitalized for acute diverticulitis needed emergency colectomy, according to a retrospective analysis of over 3000 patients.

Consensus recommendations suggest elective resection of the affected intestinal segment after three bouts of simple diverticulitis to avoid future attacks. Furthermore, early resection has been suggested for younger patients with diverticulitis as well as those who are immunocompromised. This advice is contentious since most serious diverticulitis occurs on the initial presentation and evidence for elective resection comes from tiny retrospective studies.

Percutaneous drainage of a diverticular abscess has not been linked to a higher risk of recurrence or worsening of the illness, and it does not need an elective colectomy.

Antibiotics are commonly prescribed for most patients with acute diverticulitis, but new research has cast doubt on their effectiveness, particularly in mild, uncomplicated cases. Antimicrobial treatment in acute uncomplicated diverticulitis seems to lengthen patients' hospital stays without reducing overall or individual complication rates.

- Eat a well-balanced diet that contains a broad range of foods.

- Frequently consume meals that are rich in fiber.

- Fiber may help prevent the formation of diverticula (sacs or pouches in the colon) and may make diverticular disease symptoms less severe. Diverticula that have already formed cannot be repaired with fiber.

- Vegetables and fruits should make up half of your plate.

- Whole grains with more fiber, such as whole-grain bread, noodles, brown rice, oats, and bran cereals, should be included.

- Slowly and gradually increase your intake of higher-fiber meals. Too much fiber in one sitting may induce flatulence and cramps.

- Include foods containing seeds, such as blueberries, strawberries, and tomatoes, as well as almonds, maize, and popcorn. Evidence indicates that eliminating certain foods isn't required and doesn't assist with symptom reduction.

- Protein meals should account for one-quarter of your plate. Lentils, beans, peas, tofu, fish, poultry, lean meat, nuts, seeds, and dairy are protein foods.

- Increase your consumption of lentils, beans, and peas. They are foods that are rich in fiber.

- Limit your intake of red meats like beef, pig, and lamb. According to some research, consuming a lot of red meat raises the risk of diverticular illness.

- Each day, drink 6 to 8 cups (1.5 to 2.0 L) of liquids. Make water your preferred beverage. Fiber helps to make your stools soft and easy to pass by drawing water into them.

- Exercise on a regular basis. Follow the Canadian Physical Activity Guidelines' guidelines for your age group.

Progression Of Treatment For Diverticulitis Flare-Up

When a flare-up (diverticulitis) develops, your doctor will likely suggest a restricted-fiber or fluid diet and physical rest, as well as antibiotics, antispasmodics, and pain relievers. In extreme instances, your doctor may suggest that you be admitted to the hospital for intravenous nutrition so that your gut may rest for a few days.

Medical treatment for diverticulitis may be effective, but if bouts become recurrent, surgical excision of the afflicted region may be required. Approximately 1% of people with the diverticular disease need surgery. In many instances, the surgeon may perform a colectomy (removal of the diseased section of the intestine) and reconnect the remaining ends. If this is not feasible or safe, the surgeon may move the colon's end to a new surgical hole in the abdominal wall (colostomy). After that, the patient wears a detachable device that collects the bowel contents. Depending on the conditions, a colostomy may be needed either temporarily or permanently.

Diverticular Disease Outlook

A diverticulum does not go away on its own once it has formed. A well-balanced, high-fiber diet, started as early as possible in life, seems to be the greatest preventive strategy for diverticular disease. This diet also has a number of additional health advantages. You may be able to minimize future diverticula formation and painful flare-ups by drinking enough fluids and keeping physically active. By adopting these lifestyle adjustments, many people with diverticular disease may live symptom-free. Medical and surgical therapies are available for individuals whose illness persists and does not respond to these changes.

Remedies Can Help Treat Diverticulitis

Diverticulitis is a digestive system inflammatory disease.

Diverticula are small pouches that may develop in the large intestine. Diverticulosis is the medical term for this ailment. Diverticulitis is a disease that occurs when these pouches become inflamed or infected.

Diverticulitis is a painful condition that may progress to further problems. Certain meals will frequently exacerbate a person's symptoms if they have the disease.

1. **Try a liquid diet**

A brief liquid diet may be recommended by a doctor to someone who is having a flare-up of symptoms.

The following are some liquid diet meals and beverages that may be prepared at home:

- » no fruit pulp or bits ice popsicles

- » without milk, water, coffee, and tea
- » fruit juices that have been strained to remove the pulp, such as white grape or apple juice
- » chicken or beef broth
- » soft drinks or sports drinks
- » Jell-O without fruit

A liquid diet should only be followed for as long as a doctor advises. This is to make sure they don't miss out on any important nutrients.

A doctor will suggest gradually reintroducing solid meals to the diet when the symptoms improve.

2. Adopt a low fiber diet

A low-fiber diet may also assist with the symptoms of diverticulitis.

Low-fiber foods include the following:

- » eggs
- » dairy products
- » well-cooked vegetables without seeds or skins
- » well-cooked or ground meat
- » white bread
- » white pasta
- » white rice
- » Fruits without seeds or skins, boiled or canned
- » low fiber cereals

Symptoms will typically improve after 2–4 days, following which a person may gradually introduce modest quantities of fiber back into their diet.

3. Increase fiber intake

Doctors suggest that patients with diverticulitis incorporate fiber in their diets unless they are having a symptom flare-up.

Constipation may be avoided with the use of fiber. If a person is straining to evacuate feces, the large intestine may bulge, increasing the chance of a pouch forming.

It's also crucial to drink enough water to keep your stools soft and simple to pass.

The 2015–2020 Dietary Guidelines for Americans

Fiber consumption of 14 grams per 1,000 calories is recommended by Trusted Source.

The following foods are rich in fiber:

- vegetables, including potatoes, green peas, a cabbage, and squash
- fruits, including apples, pears, avocados, and bananas
- grains, including a whole meal bread, pasta, rice, quinoa, and barley
- high fiber cereals, including bran and oats
- beans and pulses, including chickpeas, lentils, kidney beans, and split peas

4. Get more vitamin D

According to some studies, individuals with low vitamin D levels are more likely to develop diverticulitis and associated consequences. Though, this has yet to be confirmed in a subsequent study.

Vitamin D intake for adults should be 15 micrograms per day. The sections that follow will go over some of the many methods a person may get vitamin D.

FOOD SOURCES

Some food sources of vitamin D include:

- some mushrooms, including those grown under UV light
- A fatty fish, such as tuna, salmon, and mackerel
- fortified foods, such as breakfast cereals, plant milk, and margarine
- cheese
- beef liver
- eggs

Sun exposure

Sun exposure provides most individuals with a portion of their daily vitamin D need. UV radiation transforms skin molecules into vitamin D.

Vitamin D is also stored in the liver and fat cells for usage when light levels are lower.

Although sunshine aids in vitamin D production, individuals should use sunscreen and avoid tanning beds to protect themselves from sun damage.

Dietary supplements

Vitamin D may also be taken as a supplement to boost one's levels. This may be beneficial during the winter months when light levels are low. It may also benefit those who do not consume enough vitamin D-rich meals.

D-2 (ergocalciferol) and D-3 (cholecalciferol) vitamin D supplements are available (cholecalciferol). According to the National Institutes of Health, vitamin D-2 may be less effective than vitamin D-3 at larger dosages (NIH).

5. Apply a heating pad

Some people find that applying heat to their stomachs relieves their severe stomach cramps.

People may try a variety of heat pads, including:

- microwaveable heat pads
- electric heat pads
- hot water bottles

Electric equipment should be set to a low level and hot water bottles should be covered with a cloth to avoid burns.

6. Try probiotics

Probiotics are good microorganisms that reside in your intestines. They may also assist with stomach issues in certain instances.

According to a 2016 study, probiotics may help with diverticular disease symptoms and recurrence. However, there isn't enough data to say if probiotics are an effective therapy for diverticulitis just yet.

People may take a probiotic supplement or eat probiotic-rich fermented foods.

The following are some examples of fermented foods:

- » miso
- » live yogurt
- » sauerkraut
- » kefir
- » kimchi

It's a good idea to start with modest quantities of probiotics or probiotic meals when trying them for the first time. Different meals and probiotic strains are tolerated differently by different people.

Probiotics may sometimes produce unpleasant side effects, including gas, bloating, and diarrhea.

7. Get more exercise

Endorphins, the body's natural pain relievers, are released during exercise. This may assist with the discomfort caused by diverticulitis.

According to a 2019 analysis, low-to-medium impact exercise offers anti-inflammatory properties. According to the Physical Activity Guidelines for Americans, adults should receive at least 2 hours and 30 minutes of moderate-intensity exercise each week.

The American Heart Association (AHA) recommends moderate-intensity exercise in the following ways:

- » cycling (slower than 10 miles per hour)
- » gardening
- » A brisk walking (at least 2.5 miles per hour)
- » tennis
- » water aerobics
- » dancing

Exercise can also help prevent constipation.

8. **Try herbal remedies**

People with diverticulitis may benefit from herbs and spices that have anti-inflammatory or antibacterial effects.

However, since there isn't enough data on how they function in individuals with diverticulitis, it's uncertain how successful they are.

Because herbal treatments may mix with medicines, it is critical that individuals consult a doctor before starting a new product.

Herbs and spices may be consumed as a meal or as a supplement. Consider the following scenario:

- Anti-inflammatory effects of Frankincense (Boswellia serrata). Frankincense resin may be used as a supplement in tablet or tincture form.
- Allicin, one of garlic's active components, has inherent antibacterial capabilities.
- Turmeric contains the anti-inflammatory compound curcumin. It has been a long history of usage in Ayurvedic medicine, and it is available in three forms: fresh root, dried spice, and tablet.

Garlic has a high content of fermentable oligosaccharides, disaccharides, monosaccharides, and polyols, making it a good addition to meals (FODMAPs). FODMAPs are a kind of carbohydrate that, in some individuals, may cause digestive issues. A pure allicin supplement may be simpler to tolerate for these individuals.

- Nothing by Mouth

For a few hours a day, don't eat anything.

- Clear Liquid Diet

Start incorporating broth, ice pops, Jello, water, and apple juice for a few days.

- Soft Food Diet

Add yogurt, applesauce, grains, bananas, and fruit without skin as you start to feel better.

» Return to Regular Diet

Within a few days, you should feel much better. This is the time to return to a normal diet gradually.

In the Western world, diverticulitis is quite prevalent. It may usually be managed with a combination of short-term dietary modifications and medicines.

However, if problems arise, they may be very dangerous. If you have serious diverticulitis, your doctor will most likely recommend inpatient treatment. It's possible that you'll require surgery to restore the damage to your colon.

Consult your doctor if you have diverticulitis or have concerns about your risk of getting it. They can assist you in learning how to manage this illness and maintain your digestive health.

How do you manage diverticular bleeding?

Lower gastrointestinal hemorrhage is often caused by diverticular bleeding. The majority of patients report a large, painless rectal bleeding. If the bleeding is significant, the first steps in resuscitation should be airway maintenance and oxygen augmentation, followed by hemoglobin and hematocrit measurements, blood type, and cross-matching. In the case of persistent bleeding, patients may need intravenous fluid resuscitation with normal saline or lactated Ringer's solution, followed by a transfusion of packed red blood cells. In around 80% of individuals, the diverticular bleeding resolves on its own. Patients should be admitted to the critical care unit if they have serious bleeding or substantial comorbidities. Colonoscopy is the suggested first diagnostic test, which should be done within 12 to 48 hours after presenting symptoms and following a fast bowel preparation with polyethylene glycol solutions. Endoscopic therapeutic procedures may be done if the bleeding cause is detected via colonoscopy. These include epinephrine injections and electrocautery treatment. If the cause of the bleeding cannot be determined, radionuclide imaging (i.e., a technetium 99m-tagged red blood cell scan) should be done, followed by arteriography. Other treatment methods, such as selective embolization, intra-arterial vasopressin infusion, or surgery, should be explored for continuing diverticular bleeding.

What causes diverticular bleeding?

The exact reason pouches (diverticula) develop in the colon wall is unknown. Diverticula develop when high pressure within the colon presses against weak areas in the colon wall, according to doctors.

Normally, a diet high in fiber (also known as roughage) results in bulky stool that moves readily through the colon. To pass tiny, hard feces, the colon must apply greater pressure than normal if the diet is poor in fiber. A low-fiber diet may also lengthen the time feces stays in the colon, contributing to elevated blood pressure.

When high pressure presses against weak regions in the colon, pouches may develop. Blood veins penetrate through the muscular layer of the gut wall to provide blood to the inner wall, creating weak areas. When the blood artery leading to the pouch bursts, bleeding ensues.

What are the symptoms?

Diverticular hemorrhage typically results in rectum bleeding that is abrupt and severe. Blood clots may be dark crimson or brilliant red. There is usually no discomfort, and the bleeding will cease on its own.

How is diverticular bleeding diagnosed?

Other sources of bleeding must be ruled out before diverticular bleeding may be identified. A medical history and physical exam, as well as certain tests, will be performed by your doctor. To locate the source of recurrent bleeding, imaging techniques such as angiography (also known as arteriography) may be used. Colonoscopy, which involves seeing the whole large intestine (colon) using a long, flexible, lighted viewing scope (colonoscope), is considered to be one of the most effective diagnostics for determining the cause of gastrointestinal bleeding.

To find the cause of bleeding, your doctor may do a technetium-labeled red blood cell bleeding scan. A tiny quantity of radioactive substance called technetium is added to the blood in this test, and some blood is collected from you. The technetium-laced blood is then injected back into your body and tracked back to the cause of the bleeding.

How is it treated?

Diverticula bleeding usually stops on its own. If it doesn't, therapy to halt it and replenish lost blood may be required, and you may need to be admitted to the hospital. Intravenous fluids, blood transfusions, medication injections, and, in rare instances, surgery to remove the diseased portion of the colon are all possible treatments.

Can diverticular bleeding be prevented?

Diverticula may be avoided by eating a high-fiber diet, drinking enough of water, and moving frequently. If you already have diverticulosis, however, diet may not be effective in preventing bleeding.

If you use aspirin on a daily basis, you may have a greater risk of diverticular bleeding (more than 4 days a week)

Non - operative treatment of most diverticular bleeding in the elderly is generally tolerated. Treatment success and safety seem to be unaffected by prior diverticular bleeding, starting hemoglobin, or the quantity of blood transfused. The vast majority of patients are managed without surgery. The surgical procedure seems to be well tolerated.

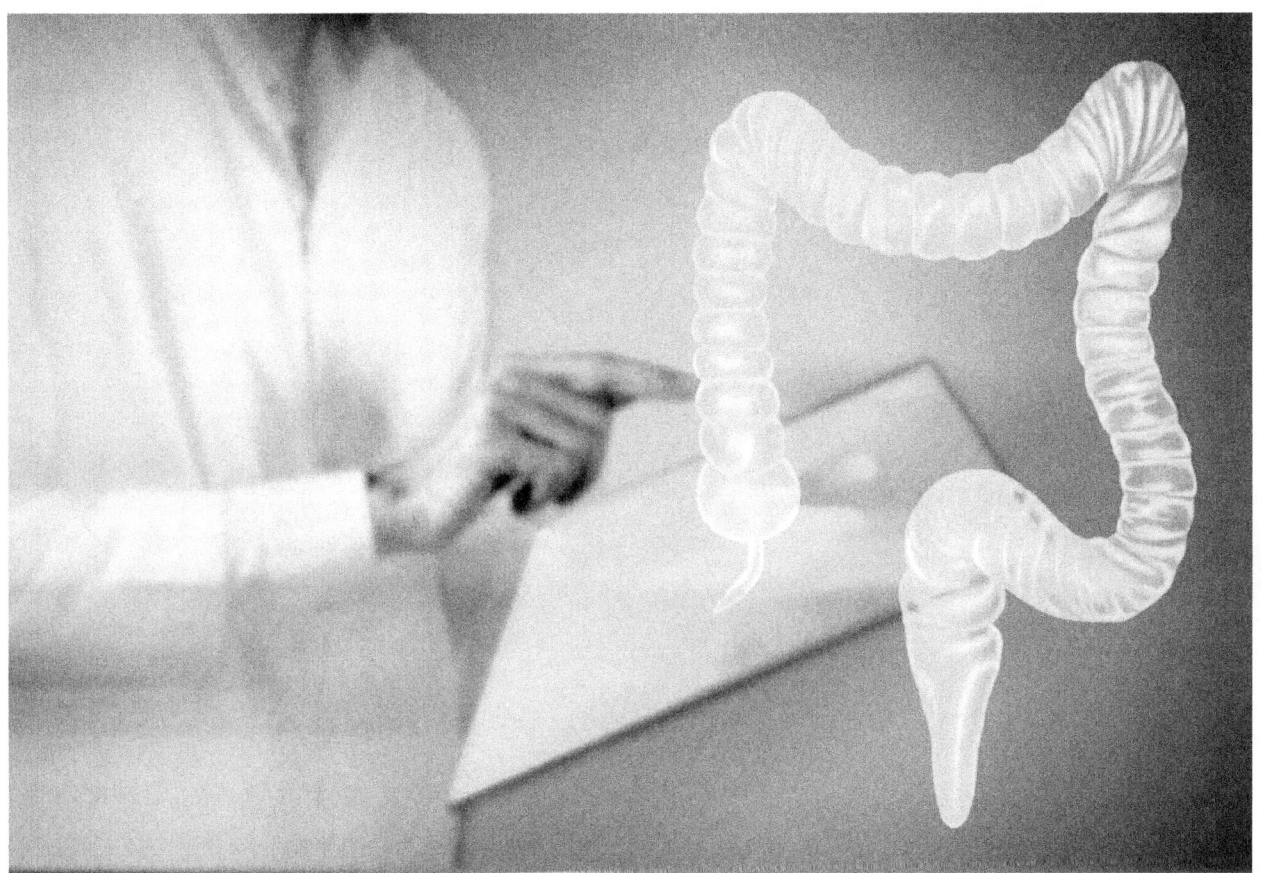

CHAPTER 3: HOW TO PREVENT DIVERTICULITIS FLARE-UPS WITH FOOD

Diverticulitis is an inflammatory disease of the digestive system. It's a diverticulosis infection. These are tiny pockets that form in the intestine's lining.

When weak areas in the intestinal wall give way under pressure, causing portions to protrude out, diverticula form. Diverticulosis is the presence of diverticula. Diverticulitis occurs when the intestines become inflamed or infected.

Diverticulosis is more common in those over the age of 50. Diverticulosis affects around 58 percent of those over 60, according to the National Institute of Diabetes and Digestive and Kidney Diseases (NIDDK). Diverticulitis is not as prevalent as it formerly was: Diverticulitis affects only around 5% of individuals with diverticulosis.

Diverticulitis may cause a variety of health issues and consequences, including:

- bloody bowel movements
- nausea
- fever
- severe abdominal pain
- fistula
- an abscess or a tissue pocket irritated

Foods To Avoid With Diverticulitis

During diverticulitis flare-ups, doctors used to suggest a low-fiber, clear liquid diet.

However, some doctors now think that if you have diverticulosis or diverticulitis, you don't have to avoid specific foods.

Diverticulitis treatment, on the other hand, is dependent on the individual. Some individuals may find that eliminating particular foods is beneficial.

During minor flare-ups, some physicians still suggest a clear liquid diet. They may suggest switching to a low-fiber diet until symptoms subside, gradually increasing to a high-fiber diet.

The sections that follow examine the evidence behind certain foods that you should avoid if you have diverticulosis or diverticulitis.

High FODMAP foods

Some patients with irritable bowel syndrome benefit from following a low FODMAP diet (IBS). Some people with diverticulitis may benefit from it as well.

FODMAPs are carbohydrate types. The list includes fermentable oligosaccharides, disaccharides, monosaccharides, and polyols.

According to some studies, a low FODMAP diet may help individuals avoid or treat diverticulitis by preventing excessive pressure in the colon.

People who follow this diet avoid foods that are rich in FODMAPS. This includes, for example, the following foods:

- Certain fruits, such as apples, pears, and plums
- legumes
- Dairy foods, such as milk, yogurt, and ice cream
- foods high in trans fats
- onions and garlic
- soy
- fermented foods, such as sauerkraut or kimchi
- cabbage
- beans
- Brussels sprouts

Red and processed meat

A diet rich in red and processed meats may raise your chance of getting diverticulitis, according to a 2018 study. A diet rich in fruits, vegetables, and whole grains may help lower the risk of heart disease.

Foods high in sugar and fat

The typical Western diet is rich in fat, sugar, and fiber but low in fiber. As a result, a person's chance of getting diverticulitis may rise.

According to a 2017 research including over 46,000 male participants.

The following foods may help prevent or decrease the symptoms of diverticulitis:

- full-fat dairy
- red meat
- refined grains
- fried food

Should I Avoid High Fiber Foods?

Fiber's impact on diverticulitis varies from person to person. In the past, physicians advised a low-fiber or clear liquid diet for patients with diverticulitis. Some physicians nowadays are no longer following this advice.

According to a 2018 study, dietary fiber may decrease the symptoms of diverticular illness and improve gastrointestinal function. According to the researchers, fiber may enhance colon health by allowing for improved stomach motility and stool bulk.

Poor fiber diets, coupled with excessive meat consumption, low physical activity, and smoking, have been linked to an increased incidence of diverticulitis in certain studies.

High fiber foods include:

- fruits
- navy beans, chickpeas, lentils, and kidney beans are examples of beans and legumes.
- vegetables
- Brown rice, quinoa, oatmeal, maize, spelled, and bulgur are examples of whole grains.

While some studies have connected a high-fiber diet to a lower incidence of diverticulitis, this may not be appropriate for someone suffering from a flare-up.

Fiber bulks up the stool and may cause painful colon spasms during a flare-up. During an acute flare, your doctor may advise you to avoid fiber.

Each individual is unique. Before making major dietary changes, it's usually a good idea to get medical advice.

Drink lots of water while adding fiber to your diet to prevent constipation.

SUMMARY

When you don't have a diverticulitis flare-up, a high-fiber diet may help maintain your gut health and decrease the likelihood of flares.

What Type Foods Should I Eat During A Diverticulitis Flare?

Your doctor may recommend specific dietary modifications to make diverticulitis more tolerable and less likely to develop over time.

If you're suffering from an acute case of diverticulitis, your doctor may recommend a low-fiber or clear liquid diet to alleviate your symptoms.

They may advise adhering to a low-fiber diet until symptoms subside, then gradually increasing to a high-fiber diet to avoid recurrent flares.

Low fiber foods

If you experience symptoms of diverticulitis, you should try eating the following low-fiber foods:

- » potatoes with no skin
- » white rice, white bread, or white pasta (however, if you're gluten-sensitive, stay away from gluten-containing meals)
- » cereals that are dry and lacking in fiber
- » fish, poultry, or eggs are examples of cooked animal proteins.
- » cooked spinach, beets, carrots, or asparagus
- » olive oil or other oils processed fruits, such as applesauce or canned peaches
- » Without the skin or seeds, yellow squash, zucchini, or pumpkin
- » fruit and vegetable juices

Clear liquid diet

A clear liquid diet is a more restricted approach to symptom relief from diverticulitis. It may be prescribed by your doctor for a limited duration.

A clear liquid diet typically consists of the following items:

- ice chips
- water
- soup broth or stock
- gelatin, such as Jell-O
- clear electrolyte drinks
- cup of tea or cup of coffee without any creams, flavors, or sweeteners

OTHER DIETARY CONSIDERATIONS

Drinking lots of water every day is beneficial whether you're on a clear liquid diet or not. This helps you stay hydrated while also supporting your digestive health.

Before making any significant dietary changes, consult your doctor.

If you're on a clear liquid diet, your doctor may suggest gradually reintroducing low-fiber items into your diet as your health improves, eventually leading to a high-fiber diet.

SUMMARY

For some people, a low-fiber or clear liquid diet may help alleviate symptoms during a diverticulitis flare.

Is There A Connection Between A High Fiber Diet And A Lower Risk Of Diverticulitis?

Even while physicians may advise avoiding high fiber foods during a flare, the National Institute of Diabetes and Digestive and Kidney Diseases (NIDDK) advises eating a high fiber diet on a daily basis to decrease the risk of acute diverticulitis.

Softer stool travels through your intestines and colon more quickly and readily because fiber softens your body's waste material.

This helps prevent the development of diverticula by lowering the pressure in your digestive tract.

Even if you don't have diverticular disease, eating a high-fiber diet may help you maintain a healthy digestive tract.

Gut bacteria, according to 2016 research, have a role in diverticular illness. Future studies are expected to support modifying gut flora via a high fiber diet and probiotic supplements, but further study is required.

SUMMARY

A high-fiber diet may help reduce diverticulitis flare-ups, according to research.

The Bottom Line

A high-fiber diet can help avoid future flare-ups if you have diverticulosis but are not experiencing an episode of diverticulitis.

A low-fiber or clear liquid diet, depending on the severity of an acute diverticulitis flare-up, may be helpful in reducing symptoms.

Consult your doctor about your dietary requirements and limitations if you have diverticulitis. It's crucial to talk about how eating may help or hurt your condition.

Ask your doctor to send you to a nutritionist if you need further help. If possible, find a healthcare practitioner who has worked with individuals who have diverticulitis.

Furthermore, keep in touch with your doctor regarding your situation. Keep in mind that diverticulitis is a chronic disease that may go unnoticed for extended periods of time.

CHAPTER 4: YES FOODS VS NO FOODS FOR EACH PHASE OF DIVERTICULITIS

ACUTE DIVERTICULITIS

- Lean Protein
- White meat poultry, white fish, plant-based proteins
- Eating low-fat meat can help you lose weight and keep you fuller for longer.

High Fiber

- Quinoa, whole grains, brown rice, fortified cereals
- Constipation is prevented by insoluble fiber, which bulks up the stool and speeds up the transit of food through the stomach and intestines.

Vegetables

- Fiber-rich fruits may help alleviate constipation and improve immunity.
- Leafy greens, peas, squash, parsnips, sweet potatoes
- Consumption of starchy vegetables will boost fiber intake, which will help with indigestion.
- Pears, apples, oranges, prunes
- Fruit

Healthy Fats

Fat is a biological requirement that boosts hormone synthesis, improves nutrient absorption, and boosts heart and brain health.

Avocado, nut butter, and extra virgin olive oil

Food to Avoid:

- Seeds
- Poppy seeds, chia seeds, flax seeds, and sesame seeds have all been known to become trapped in

the diverticula. Fruit-containing seeds, such as strawberries, raspberries, and blackberries, should be avoided.

Raw vegetables
- » Because the insoluble fiber in vegetables is completely intact, they may be more difficult to digest, causing pain and discomfort. Cooking your veggies makes it easier for your body to break down fiber.

Corn
- » Corn's fiber and sugar levels induce stomach pain, resulting in digestive system inflammation.

Spicy foods

Spicy meals may cause intestinal irritation, which can result in vomiting and diarrhea. It's advisable to avoid these meals if you don't want your diverticulitis symptoms to become worse.

Cruciferous Vegetables

Broccoli, cabbage, and artichokes, for example, are rich in fiber and may be difficult to digest. It's possible that eating them may induce bloating and gas.

Milk Products

Lactose may be difficult to digest in those who have diverticulitis. Even those who aren't lactose intolerant can experience bloating, gas, and inflammation after consuming dairy products, including milk, cheese, and yogurt.

Greasy, High Fat, Fast Food

Fried food has a lot of fat, which stimulates the digestive system and promotes inflammation, leading to acid reflux, which may aggravate diverticulitis symptoms.

Excessive Alcohol

Drinking a lot of alcohol raises your chances of getting diverticulitis by 2-3 times. Due to reduced intestinal motility, scientists believe the disease is related to alcohol.

Recovery Phase

Foods to eat

Again, this is a subjective list, and anything on it may trigger you. However, these meals are often kind to diverticulitis sufferers' intestines.

If you have trouble digesting cereals and rice, try quick oatmeal, pasta or noodles, whole wheat bread, muffins, or wraps instead.

Eggs and delicate pieces of meat (such as shredded chicken, baked fish, and ground beef) are often simple to digest.

If the skin of cooked fruits and vegetables irritates you, you may need to remove it.

Potatoes and other starchy foods: It's good for your colon if you eat a lot of starch (however, you may consider peeling the potatoes first).

Water, tea, and juice: To avoid irritating your intestines, keep your juice pulp-free (like apple, grape, or cranberry instead of orange).

Foods to stay away from

Physicians used to advise patients with diverticulitis to avoid nuts, seeds, and corn products, but today they understand that such limits don't have to be given to all patients. Many individuals can consume these meals without difficulty.

Foods that may be harmful to your health

You may be able to consume these foods if you eat them cautiously, rarely, or in little amounts—or they could be too much of a colon trigger. If that's the case, you're not alone; these are the foods most likely to cause a diverticulitis flare-up.

- » **Foods that are tough to chew:** Foods that are difficult to break down are more likely to become stuck in your colon's pockets.
- » **Sunflower seeds:** for example, may be difficult to digest; strawberries seeds, on the other hand, are generally not (but they may still irritate you!).
- » **Popcorn and corn on the cob:** These meals are more prone to create problems since you consume them fast rather than chewing them thoroughly.
- » **Red meat:** Some research suggests that red meat may lead to diverticulitis flare-ups; one study published in Gut in 2018 found that males who ate more red meat than other kinds of protein, such as chicken and fish, had more attacks.

- » **High-FODMAP foods:** Some experts believe that eating a low-FODMAP diet may lower colon pressure and decrease the frequency of acute episodes that a diverticulitis patient may experience.

Prevention Phase

- » Broccoli, carrots, other root vegetables
- » Foods that are anti-inflammatory, such as avocado and olive oil
- » Apples, bananas, pears
- » Nuts and seeds
- » Oats, rye, barley, whole grains
- » Psyllium husks or fiber supplements
- » Brown rice
- » Water

Non-Compliant Foods

- » Soy
- » Beans, legumes
- » Red meat
- » Bran
- » Trans fats
- » Full-fat dairy
- » Brussels sprouts, cabbage
- » Fermented foods
- » Fried foods
- » Garlic, onions

Food Lists For Diverticulitis Diets

The diverticulitis diet is designed to help your digestive system recover and restore its health. To alleviate the symptoms, you'll decrease your fiber intake at first, then gradually raise it when your symptoms improve over the course of a few days.

Clear liquids, low-fiber foods, and high-fiber foods are the three stages:

Stage 1: Clear Liquids (~1-2 days)

- Tea or coffee without sweeteners
- Ice chips or ice pops
- Broth, preferably low in sodium
- Fruit juices
- Ice cream or milkshakes
- Water
- Gelatin
- Pudding

Stage 2: Low-Fiber/Low-Residue Foods (~2-3 days)

- Fruit or vegetable juice (no pulp)
- White bread
- Potatoes
- Low-fiber cereals
- Dairy (milk, yogurt, cheese)
- Peeled and cooked or canned vegetables/fruits
- White rice
- Fish, chicken, and eggs

Stage 3: High-Fiber Diet

- Popcorn

- Fruits and vegetables with skin
- Beets
- Psyllium powder
- Oats
- Beans
- Whole wheat and whole-grain foods
- Nuts (peanuts, Brazil nuts, etc.)
- Sesame, chia, hemp seeds
- Brown rice

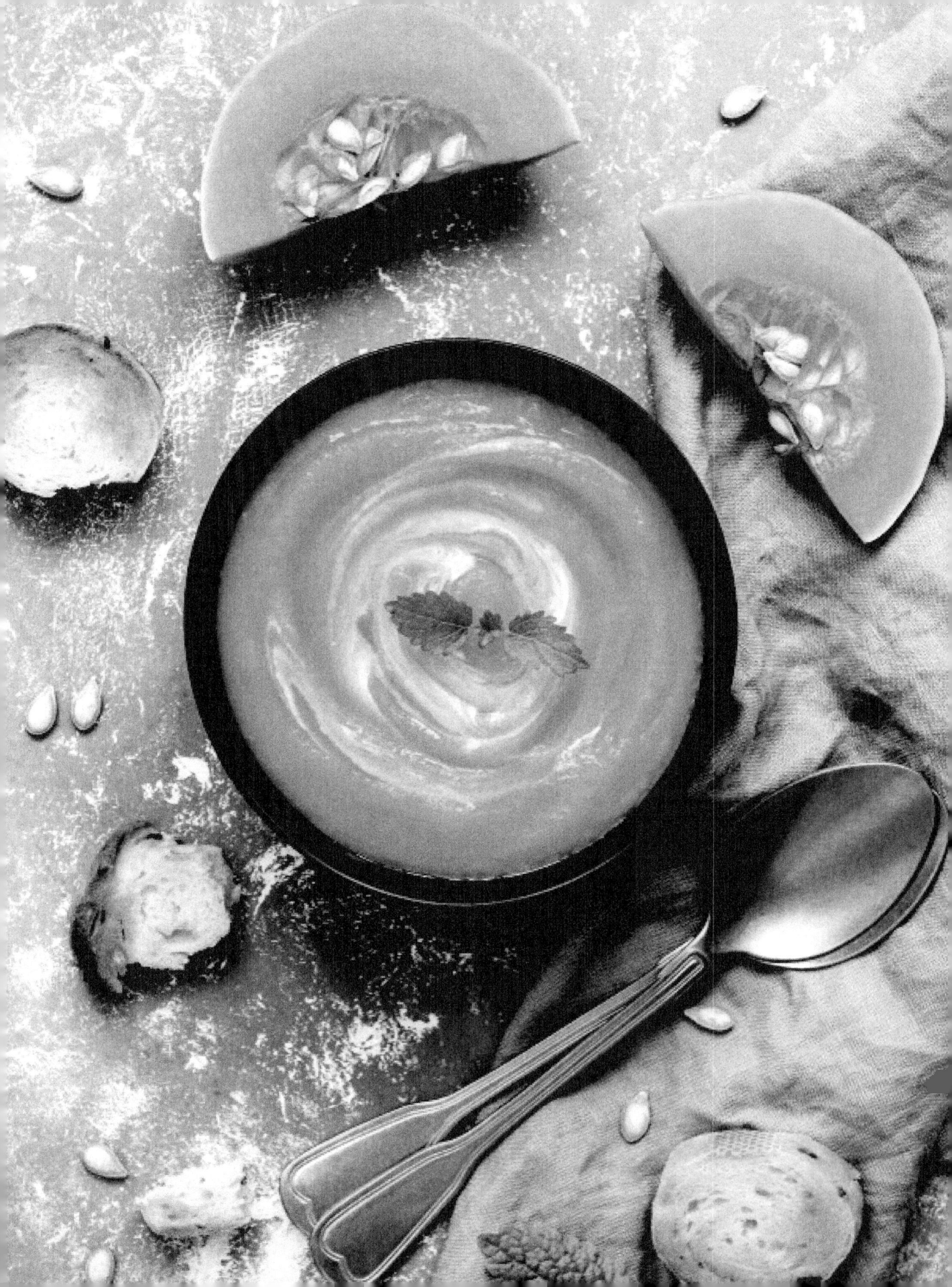

CHAPTER 5: BREAKFAST (CLEAR FLUIDS)

1. APPLE AND PEAR PITA POCKETS

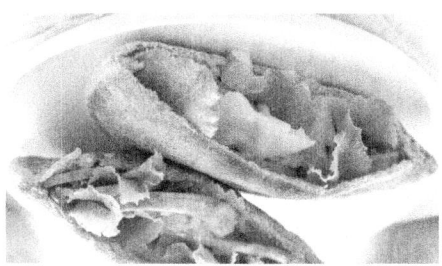

Prep Time: 10 minutes
Cook Time: 10 minutes
Total Time: 20 minutes
Servings: 2
Ingredients::
- 1/2 of small apple, unpeeled, chopped
- ½ of a small pear, unpeeled, chopped
- 1/4 of Cup cottage cheese
- One whole-wheat pita bread

Directions:
1. In a mixing bowl, combine the apple, pear, and cottage cheese.
2. To make a pocket, slice the pita bread in half. Place the fruit mixture in the pocket.
3. For extra sweetness, add a pinch of cinnamon or a drizzle of honey or agave syrup.
4. It makes 20 mini pitas halves

Nutrition Facts: Calories: 67 | Carbohydrates: 12 g | Protein: 2 g | Fat: 2 g | Cholesterol: 86 mg

2. BRANDY JAVA ICE

Prep Time: 2 minutes
Cook Time: 2 minutes
Total Time: 4 minutes
Servings: 2

Ingredients:
- Four scoops of vanilla ice cream large
- 2 oz brandy
- Two teaspoons of ground coffee, not instant granules

Directions:
1. In a blender, combine all of the ingredients and blend until smooth. Enjoy!

Nutrition Facts: Calories: 339 | Carbohydrates: 21 g | Protein: 5 g | Fat: 15 g | Cholesterol: 100 mg

3. APPLE RAISIN PANCAKES

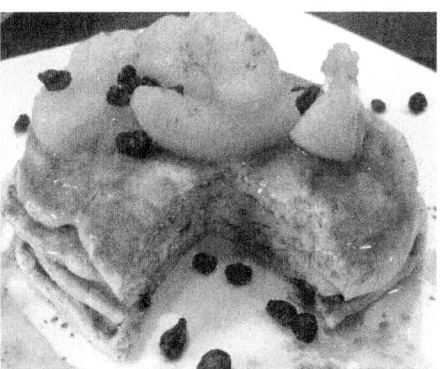

Prep Time: 10 minutes
Cook Time: 30 minutes
Total Time: 40 minutes
Servings: 4

Ingredients:
- Two eggs
- One Cup unsweetened applesauce
- One Teaspoon cinnamon
- Two Teaspoons brown sugar
- One Cup wheat flour
- ½ Cup white flour
- Two Teaspoons baking powder

- Two Teaspoons vanilla
- ½ Cup golden, seedless raisins
- Non-stick cooking spray

Directions:
1. Whisk the eggs in a medium mixing basin until light and frothy.
2. Stir in the applesauce, cinnamon, sugar, flours, baking powder, vanilla, and raisins until smooth.
3. Over medium heat, heat a griddle or a pan. We are using nonstick frying spray, coat the pan. Pour approximately 1/4 cup of batter each pancake onto a heated pan.
4. Cook until the pancakes' edges begin to boil. Cook until golden on the other side. If desired, top the pancakes with more applesauce.

Nutrition Facts: Calories: 55 | Carbohydrates: 10 g | Protein: 13 g | Fat: 1 g | Cholesterol: 10 mg

- 1/4 - 1/2 cup buckwheat flour (or plain flour)
- 1/4 cup blueberries
- pinch of cinnamon (optional)
- One tablespoon coconut oil for frying

Directions:
1. After mashing the bananas, add the flour and cinnamon.
2. Stir in the blueberries until they are evenly distributed.
3. Heat the coconut oil in a nonstick frying pan over high heat.
4. Reduce the heat to medium-low and pour one tablespoon of batter into the frying pan for each fritter.
5. Fry fritters until both sides are golden brown.
6. Remove the fritters from the pan and set them aside to cool slightly before serving.

Nutrition Facts: Calories: 62 | Carbohydrates: 13 g | Protein: 1 g | Fat: 2 g | Cholesterol: 18 mg

4. BANANA AND BLUEBERRY FRITTERS

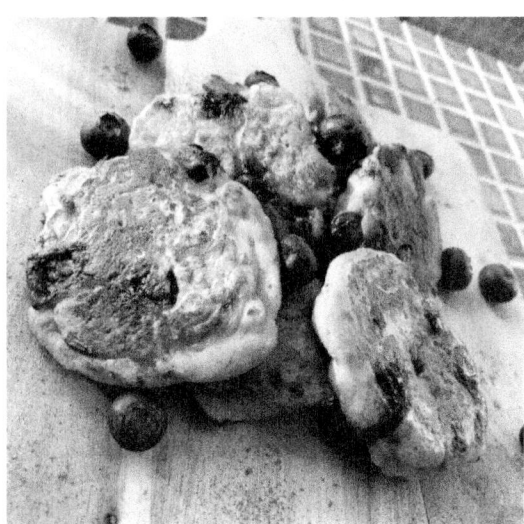

Prep Time: 10 minutes
Cook Time: 5 minutes
Total Time: 15 minutes
Servings: 6
Ingredients:
- Two ripe bananas

5. BANANA AND OAT COOKIES

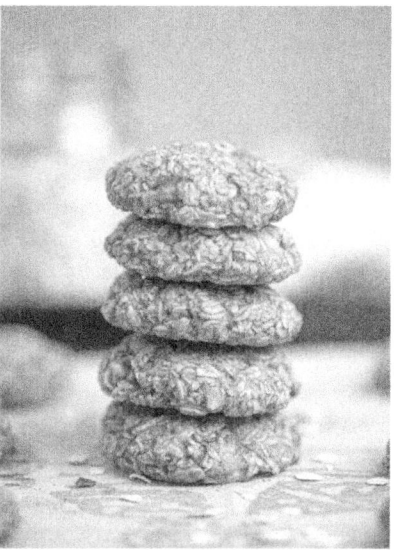

Prep Time: 10 minutes
Cook Time: 15 minutes
Total Time: 25 minutes
Servings: 15
Ingredients:
- 2 Ripe bananas

- 165g 1 3/4 cup Oats

Directions:
1. Preheat the oven to 180°C (350°F)/Gas Mark 4 and line a baking tray/sheet with parchment or baking paper.
2. Mash the bananas well in a large mixing basin until smooth. Mix in the oats until they are completely mixed.
3. To taste, add any other ingredients
4. Form tablespoon-sized cookies and put them on a baking sheet lined with parchment paper. (Be careful to create cookie forms rather than balls, since they won't expand into shape like regular cookies)
5. Bake for about 15 minutes, or until golden brown and firm.
6. Allow time for the food to cool before eating.

Nutrition Facts: Calories: 55 | Carbohydrates: 11 g | Protein: 1 g | Fat: 1 g | Cholesterol: 11 mg

6. BANANA PANCAKES

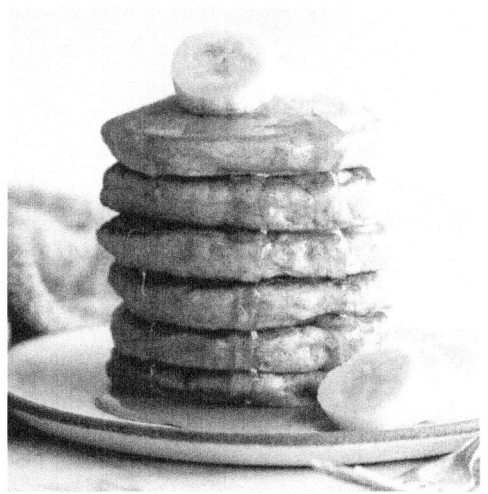

Prep Time: 5 minutes
Cook Time: 5 minutes
Total Time: 10 minutes
Servings: 14

Ingredients:
- One large of ripe banana
- Two eggs
- 3/4 tablespoon of cinnamon (optional)
- 1/2 tablespoon of Coconut Oil (or butter)

Directions:
1. In a mixing bowl, mash the banana.
2. Combine the eggs and mix well.
3. Stir in the cinnamon (if desired) or other flavorings.
4. In a frying pan, melt the coconut oil (or butter) over medium heat.
5. To create one pancake, pour one tablespoon batter onto the pan. Fill the pan to the top, allowing enough room to flip each pancake effortlessly.
6. Cook for Two minutes on each side. Take care while flipping the pancakes since they are extremely fragile.
7. Serve with a choice of toppings.

Nutrition Facts: Calories: 21 | Carbohydrates: 2 g | Protein: 2 g | Fat: 1 g | Cholesterol: 23 mg

7. SWEET POTATO PANCAKES

Prep Time: 5 minutes
Cook Time: 12 minutes
Total Time: 17 minutes
Servings: 13

Ingredients:
- 125 gram (1/2 cup) of Sweet Potato Puree and Mashed Sweet Potato
- Two eggs
- 3/4 tablespoon ground cinnamon (optional)
- 1/4 tablespoon ground ginger (optional)
- One tablespoon coconut oil (for frying)

Directions:
1. Whisk the eggs and sweet potato together in a large mixing basin until thoroughly combined. Stir in the cinnamon and ginger (if using) until well combined.
2. Heat the oil in a frying pan over medium heat.
3. Spoon one spoonful of the mixture into the pan (little pancakes work best) and continue until the pan is completely filled.
4. Reduce the heat to medium/low and continue to cook for an additional 2 to 3 minutes.

5. Cook until done on the other side (approx 2-3 mins)
6. Repeat till you've used up all of the mixtures.

Nutrition Facts: Calories: 21 | Carbohydrates: 2 g | Protein: 1 g | Fat: 1 g | Cholesterol: 25 mg

8. LENTIL SPINACH PANCAKES

Prep Time: 5 minutes
Cook Time: 10 minutes
Total Time: 15 minutes
Servings: 14

Ingredients:
- 180g (1 cup) Red Split Lentils
- 1/3 cup Water
- One Garlic Clove, minced
- One Carrot, grated
- 1/4 tablespoon Ground Cumin
- 1/2 tablespoon Smoked Paprika
- Two handfuls of Baby Spinach (finely chopped into ribbons)
- Two tablespoon Fresh Lemon Juice
- 1/4 tablespoon Salt*
- One tablespoon Oil (for frying)

Directions:
1. Cover the lentils with water in a mixing dish. Allow soaking for at least one night.
2. Drain the lentils and combine them with the water in a blender or food processor. Blend until the batter is smooth. You may discover that you need to add additional water; if so, do so.)
3. Heat 1/2 tablespoon of the oil in a frying pan over medium-high heat. Reduce the heat to medium-low and sauté the carrot, garlic, smoked paprika, cumin, and spinach until softened (around 4-5 mins).
4. Combine the lentil batter, the sautéed veggies, and the lemon juice in a large mixing basin.
5. Over medium-high heat, heat a nonstick frying pan. Add a sprinkle of oil when the pan is heated (or alternatively, use spray oil). Place a spoonful of batter in the pan and spread it out with the back of your spoon (to make them thinner). To fill the pan, repeat the process.
6. Cook each side for at least 2 minutes (this will vary depending on the pan, heat and how thin your pancake is). Look for bubbles to develop, and your pancakes should be able to be easily flipped.
7. Remove the pancakes from the pan and continue with the rest of the batter. Serve

Nutrition Facts: Calories: 58 | Carbohydrates: 9 g | Protein: 4 g | Fat: 1 g | Cholesterol: 19 mg

9. CHICKPEA PANCAKES RECIPE

Prep Time: 10 minutes
Cook Time: 15 minutes
Total Time: 25 minutes
Servings: 23

Ingredients:
- 1 cup (120g) Chickpea Flour
- 1 ½ cups 375ml Water
- Two tablespoons of Olive Oil *See Note 1
- 1 Carrot, finely grated
- 1/4 Red Capsicum, finely chopped
- 1 Spring Onion, finely chopped
- 1/4 tablespoon Turmeric
- 1/4 tablespoon Cumin
- Two tablespoons of Chopped Coriander (cilantro)
- 1/4 tablespoon Salt

Directions:
1. Combine the chickpea flour and water in a mixing basin, constantly stirring to create a smooth, lump-free batter. Set aside.

2. Heat 1/2 tablespoon of the oil in a frying pan over medium-high heat. Combine the carrot, onion, turmeric, and cumin in a mixing bowl. Reduce the heat to medium-low and continue to simmer until the vegetables are softened (around 4-5 mins)
3. Combine the carrot mixture, chopped coriander, and salt in the chickpea batter (if using). Stir until everything is well mixed.
4. Over medium-high heat, heat a nonstick frying pan. When the pan is heated, pour in the olive oil (or alternatively, use spray oil). Place a tablespoon of batter in the pan and spread it out with the back of your spoon (to make them thinner). To fill the pan, repeat the process. (*Please see Note 3)
5. Cook each side for at least 2 minutes (this will vary depending on the pan, heat and how thin your pancake is). Look for bubbles to develop (as seen above), and your pancakes should be able to be easily flipped.
6. Remove the pancakes from the pan and repeat the process with the remaining batter.

Nutrition Facts: Calories: 32 | Carbohydrates: 3 g | Protein: 1 g | Fat: 1 g | Cholesterol: 27 mg

10. VEGGIE CHICKPEA STICKS

Prep Time: 10 minutes
Cook Time: 15 minutes
Total Time: 25 minutes
Servings: 6

Ingredients:
- 55 g (1/2 cup) grated carrots
- Two tablespoon Chia
- 400 g can Chickpeas (drained and washed)
- One tablespoon cream cheese
- 60 (1/2 cup) grated cheddar cheese
- One tablespoon Olive Oil
- One handful of spinach leaves (chopped)
- 60 g (1/2 cup) frozen peas
- 1/2 tablespoon smoked paprika
- 1/2 tablespoon mixed dried herbs

Directions:
1. Preheat oven to 180°C/350°F/Gas 4 and line two baking pans with reusable baking sheets.
2. Squeeze as much juice as possible from the carrots. Reserving the carrot juice, add water to produce a total of 80ml (1/3 cup) liquid.
3. Set aside the chia and carrot juice combination.
4. In a mixing bowl, combine all of the remaining ingredients and mix until smooth. Add the chia mixture and pulse until well combined.
5. Form a finger out of about a third of a spoonful of the mixture (alternatively, you could make cookie shape or nuggets). Repeat until the mixture is completed.
6. Bake for 15 minutes.

Nutrition Facts: Calories: 139 | Carbohydrates: 5 g | Protein: 8 g | Fat: 6 g | Cholesterol: 31 mg

11. APRICOT HONEY OATMEAL

Prep Time: 5 minutes
Cook Time: 5 minutes
Total Time: 10 minutes
Servings: 1

Ingredients:
- 1 Cup water or milk or almond milk
- 1/4 Cup dried apricots, chopped
- 1/2 Cup rolled oats
- 1 Tablespoon honey
- 1/4 Teaspoon cinnamon

Directions:
1. In a microwave-safe dish, combine the water or milk, apricots, honey, cinnamon, and oats.
2. Cook for about 2 minutes, stirring periodically until most of the liquid has been absorbed.

Nutrition Facts: Calories: 345 | Carbohydrates: 1 g | Protein: 29 g | Fat: 9 g | Cholesterol: 105 mg

12. ASPARAGUS AND BEAN FRITTATA

Prep Time: 20 minutes
Cook Time: 30 minutes
Total Time: 50 minutes
Servings: 4

Ingredients:
- Two Tablespoons olive oil
- One cup of chopped onion
- One minced garlic clove
- 14 oz drained and washed red, black, or white beans
- Four eggs 1 cup cooked and chopped asparagus
- a half teaspoon of salt
- 1/4 cup grated Parmesan

Directions:
1. Preheat the oven to 350°F.
2. One tablespoon olive oil, heated in a large oven-proof pan over medium-high heat Cook until the onions, garlic, and red beans are tender (about 10 minutes). Place aside.
3. In a nice medium mixing bowl, combine eggs, salt, and asparagus; set aside.
4. Pour in the egg mixture and the remaining one tablespoon olive oil into the vegetable pan. Reduce the heat to medium-low and simmer for 10 to 15 minutes, or until the mixture is set and gently browned on the bottom.
5. Sprinkle the Parmesan cheese on top of the mixture and broil for 3 to 5 minutes, or until the cheese is lightly browned and the eggs are cooked through.

Nutrition Facts: Calories: 446 | Carbohydrates: 2 g | Protein: 43 g | Fat: 29 g | Cholesterol: 215 mg

13. CHOCOLATE SMOOTHIE

Prep Time: 5 minutes
Cook Time: 0 minutes
Total Time: 5 minutes
Servings: 2

Ingredients:
- Two scoops of chocolate-flavored whey protein
- Two cups of ice
- Two tablespoons Southern Comfort® liqueur (optional)
- ½ cup evaporated milk
- ¼ cup condensed milk
- ¼ teaspoon ground cinnamon
- Pinch of nutmeg

Directions:
1. In a neat blender, combine all ingredients except the cinnamon and mix on high for 1–2 minutes, or until smooth.
2. To serve, top with whipped cream and sprinkle with cinnamon.

Nutrition Facts: Calories: 142 | Carbohydrates: 17 g | Protein: 10 g | Fat: 4 g | Cholesterol: 120 mg

14. ORANGE AND CINNAMON BISCOTTI

Prep Time: 10 minutes
Cook Time: 0 minutes
Total Time: 10 minutes
Servings: 6

Ingredients:
- 1 cup sugar
- ½ cup unsalted butter, room temperature
- Two large eggs
- Two teaspoons grated orange peel
- One teaspoon vanilla extract
- Two cups all-purpose flour
- One teaspoon cream of tartar
- ½ teaspoon baking soda
- One teaspoon ground cinnamon
- ¼ teaspoon salt

Directions:
1. Preheat the oven to 325 degrees Fahrenheit.
2. Two baking sheets, sprayed with nonstick cooking spray

3. In a large mixing basin, combine the sugar and unsalted butter until thoroughly combined.
4. Add eggs one at a time, and mix thoroughly after each addition.
5. Mix in the orange peel and vanilla extract.
6. In a medium-sized mixing bowl, combine the flour, cream of tartar, baking soda, cinnamon, and salt.
7. Combine dry ingredients with butter mixture until everything is thoroughly mixed.
8. Cut the dough in half. Place one half on a prepared baking sheet. Form each half into a log shape 3 inches broad by three-quarters of an inch high using lightly floured hands. Bake for 35 minutes or until the dough logs are firm to the touch.
9. Take the dough logs out of the oven and put them aside to cool for 10 minutes.
10. Move logs to the work surface. Using a serrated knife, cut into 12-inch-thick slices on the diagonal. Place baking sheets cut side down on a baking sheet.
11. Bake for 12 minutes, or until the bottoms are brown.
12. Bake until the bottoms of the biscotti are brown, about twelve minutes more.
13. Place on a wire rack to cool before serving.

Nutrition Facts: Calories: 139 | Carbohydrates: 33 g | Protein: 2 g | Fat: 6 g | Cholesterol: 27 mg

15. **BANANA BRAN MUFFINS**

Prep Time: 10 minutes
Cook Time: 30 minutes
Total Time: 40 minutes
Servings: 12

Ingredients:
- 1 ½ cup All-Bran cereal
- 2/3 Cups milk
- Four eggs
- 1/4 cup canola oil
- 1 cup ripe banana, mashed (about two bananas)
- 1/2 cup brown sugar
- 1 cup whole wheat flour
- Two teaspoons baking powder
- 1/2 teaspoon salt

Directions:
1. Preheat the oven to 400°F.
2. Set aside All-Bran cereal and milk in a large mixing dish. Combine the eggs, oil, mashed banana, and brown sugar on a large mixing plate.
3. In a separate mixing bowl, whisk together the flour, baking powder, and salt. Stir in the dry ingredients until barely mixed with the banana mixture.
4. Bake 15 to 18 minutes, or until golden-brown and firm, in 12 greased or paper-lined muffin pans. Allow cooling completely before serving.

Nutrition Facts: Calories: 155 | Carbohydrates: 4 g | Protein: 18 g | Fat: 4 g | Cholesterol: 172 mg

16. **BANANA BREAKFAST SMOOTHIE**

Prep Time: 10 minutes
Cook Time: 5 minutes
Total Time: 15 minutes
Servings: 1

Ingredients:
- One medium banana
- 1 cup milk, almond or regular
- 1/2 cup plain yogurt
- 1/4 Cup 100% Bran flakes
- One teaspoon vanilla extract
- Two teaspoons honey or agave syrup
- 1/2 cup ice
- One Pinch cinnamon
- One Pinch nutmeg

Directions:
1. In a neat blender, combine all of the ingredients and mix on medium speed until smooth.
2. Garnish with cinnamon and/or nutmeg if desired.

Nutrition Facts: Calories: 58 | Carbohydrates: 2 g | Protein: 3 g | Fat: 5 g | Cholesterol: 16 mg

17. SWEET & NUTTY BARS

Prep Time: 15 minutes
Cook Time: 30 minutes
Total Time: 45 minutes
Servings: 3

Ingredients:
- 2½ cups rolled oats, toasted
- ½ cup almonds
- ½ cup flax
- ½ cup peanut butter
- 1 cup dried cherries, blueberries or Craisins®
- ½ cup honey

Directions:
1. To toast the oats, place rolled oats on a baking sheet and bake for 10 minutes, or until golden brown.
2. Combine all of the ingredients in a large mixing bowl and stir until well mixed.
3. Press the protein mixture into a 9" × 9" pan that has been lightly oiled. Wrap in plastic wrap and place in the refrigerator for at least one hour or overnight.
4. Serve protein bars cut into appropriate squares.

Nutrition Facts: Calories: 283 | Carbohydrates: 39 g | Protein: 7 g | Fat: 14 g | Cholesterol: 125 mg

18. HOMEMADE HERBED BISCUITS

Prep Time: 15 minutes
Cook Time: 0 minutes
Total Time: 15 minutes
Servings: 4

Ingredients:
- 1¾ cups all-purpose flour
- One teaspoon cream of tartar
- ½ teaspoon baking soda
- ¼ cup mayonnaise
- ⅔ cup skim milk
- Three tablespoons chives or any other herb, fresh or dry to taste
- Nonstick cooking spray

Directions:
1. Preheat the oven to 400 degrees (200 degrees Celsius). Next, coat a cookie sheet with nonstick cooking spray.
2. In a large mixing basin, combine the flour, cream of tartar, and baking soda. Then, using a fork, stir in the mayonnaise until the mixture resembles coarse cornmeal.
3. Combine the milk and herbs in a separate bowl, then add to the flour mixture. Stir until everything is incorporated.
4. Place the heaping teaspoons of the mixture on the cookie sheet. 10 minutes in the oven
5. Place in the refrigerator until ready to use.

Nutrition Facts: Calories: 109 | Carbohydrates: 15 g | Protein: 3 g | Fat: 4 g | Cholesterol: 152 mg

19. SPINACH VEGETABLE BARLEY BEAN SOUP

Prep Time: 20 minutes
Cook Time: 60 minutes
Total Time: 80 minutes
Servings: 6

Ingredients:
- One tablespoon extra-virgin olive oil
- Two stalks of celery chopped
- One medium onion diced
- Two carrots chopped
- One medium leek white and pale green parts only washed thoroughly and thinly sliced
- One cup quick-cooking barley
- One tablespoon tomato paste
- 8 cups low sodium vegetable broth
- 15 oz cannellini beans or other beans rinsed and drained
- Two teaspoon sprigs of fresh thyme or one dried thyme
- One teaspoon stem fresh basil or one dried thyme
- Four handfuls of baby spinach

Directions:

1. In a soup saucepan, heat the oil. Cook until the celery, onion, carrots, and leeks are cooked, about 5 minutes, over medium heat. Cook, constantly tossing, until the barley and tomato paste are covered and glossy, approximately 30 seconds. Bring the broth, beans, thyme, and basil to a boil. Simmer for 1 hour on low heat.
2. Cook until the spinach is barely wilted (if you use Swiss chard or kale, it will take slightly longer to cook). Take off the thyme branch and the wilted basil. Season with salt and taste.

Nutrition Facts: Calories: 277 | Carbohydrates: 47 g | Protein: 14 g | Fat: 5 g | Cholesterol: 221 mg

20. SCD SOUR CREAM RECIPE

Prep Time: 5 minutes
Cook Time: 10 minutes
Total Time: 15 minutes
Servings: 2

Ingredients:
- 2 cups organic heavy cream
- 1/4 cup plain yogurt containing Lactobacillus bulgaricus L. acidophilus and S. thermophilus

Directions:
1. In a medium pan, heat cream until it reaches a simmer, around 180 degrees Fahrenheit.
2. Allow it to cool to room temperature (I let it cool down to 80 degrees).
3. Transfer 1/2 cup of the chilled cream to a mixing dish and whisk in the yogurt until well combined. Stir into the pot until well combined. Divide the milk among the mason jars.
4. Set the dehydrator to 105 degrees Fahrenheit. Allow for a 24-hour period of inactivity. Remove from the oven and place in the refrigerator until ready to eat.
5. Consume within two weeks.

Nutrition Facts: Calories: 98 | Carbohydrates: 2 g | Protein: 6 g | Fat: 7 g | Cholesterol: 98 mg

21. SKINNY PUMPKIN SPICE CHAI LATTE RECIPE

Prep Time: 5 minutes
Cook Time: 30 minutes
Total Time: 35 minutes
Servings: 3

Ingredients:
- 1-star anise
- 12 whole cloves
- 1/8 teaspoon ground allspice
- Two three-inch sticks of cinnamon
- One green cardamon pod cracked open
- One cup of water
- Four cups unsweetened non-dairy milk
- Four black tea bags I used English breakfast tea
- 1/2 cup pureed pumpkin
- 1/4 cup maple syrup
- Two tablespoons double vanilla extract
- lightly whipped cream or cashew cream optional

Directions:
1. In a small saucepan, combine star anise, whole cloves, allspice, cinnamon sticks, green cardamom pod, and water. Bring to a boil, then turn off the heat and put aside, covered, for 20 minutes.
2. Bring nondairy milk to a boil in a saucepan; remove from heat and stir in tea bags, pumpkin, maple syrup, and vanilla. Allow to steep for 10 minutes, covered. Pour into serving cups. If preferred, top with whipped cream or cashew cream.

Nutrition Facts: Calories: 137 | Carbohydrates: 23 g | Protein: 2 g | Fat: 4 g | Cholesterol: 36 mg

22. EASY TOMATO BASIL SOUP

Prep Time: 5 minutes
Cook Time: 10 minutes
Total Time: 15 minutes
Servings: 4

Ingredients:
- One teaspoon of olive oil is optional; you can use a drop of water to sauté instead to keep the recipe oil-free
- One medium of onion chopped
- Three large cloves of garlic were sliced very finely, so used four but adjust to suit your tastes
- Seven cups / 1400 g of chopped fresh tomatoes
- One handful of basil leaves and stalks are fine
- Two teaspoons of salt adjust to taste

Directions:
1. Heat the oil or a couple of tablespoons of water in a pan over medium heat.
2. When the oil is heated, add the onions and garlic and sauté for a couple of minutes, or until they begin to turn golden.
3. Toss in the diced tomatoes. Cook, occasionally turning, over medium heat until the tomatoes have broken down and become mushy.
4. Remove from the heat, then add the basil, salt, and blitz in a blender or with a stick immersion blender until smooth.
5. Serve right away.

Nutrition Facts: Calories: 78 | Carbohydrates: 28 g | Protein: 4 g | Fat: 1 g | Cholesterol: 17 mg

23. SUGAR-FREE CHOCOLATE MOUSSE

Prep Time: 10 minutes
Cook Time: 35 minutes
Total Time: 45 minutes
Servings: 2

Ingredients:
- One avocado pitted and peeled
- 1/4 cup unsweetened cocoa powder
- 1/2 cup unsweetened almond milk
- One teaspoon vanilla extract
- 1/8 teaspoon salt
- 1/4 teaspoon liquid vanilla or chocolate stevia
- non-dairy whipped topping optional

Directions:
1. In a high-powered mixing bowl or blender, combine all of the ingredients and mix until totally smooth. If desired, top with whipped topping.

Nutrition Facts: Calories: 146 | Carbohydrates: 11 g | Protein: 13 g | Fat: 12 g | Cholesterol: 113 mg

24. BLUEBERRY SMOOTHIE

Prep Time: 5 minutes
Cook Time: 0 minutes
Total Time: 5 minutes
Servings: 2

Ingredients:
- 1 cup of unsweetened vanilla almond milk
- 1 cup of frozen blueberries
- ¾ cup of frozen banana coins (~1 medium ripe banana)
- Two tablespoons of almond or peanut butter

Directions:
1. **The night before:** Peel the banana and chopped it into coins. The night before making this smoothie, place the coins in a sealed bag in the freezer.
2. **On the day of** In a large, strong blender, combine the almond milk (see Note 1), frozen blueberries, frozen banana, and almond butter. Blend until smooth. Adjust the seasoning to taste. (Depending on the sweetness of the banana, you may need to add some honey or maple syrup; we generally don't!)
3. Enjoy right now.

Nutrition Facts: Calories: 416 | Carbohydrates: 54 g | Protein: 10 g | Fat: 22 g | Cholesterol: 16 mg

25. KATZ'S MAGIC MINERAL BROTH

Prep Time: 20 minutes
Cook Time: 120 minutes
Total Time: 140 minutes
Servings: 4

Ingredients:
- Three unpeeled organic carrots cut into thirds
- One unpeeled medium organic yellow onion cut into chunks
- One organic leek both white and green parts rinsed well, cut into thirds
- 1/2 bunch organic celery including the heart, cut into thirds
- Three cloves unpeeled organic garlic halved
- 1/2 bunch fresh flat-leaf organic parsley
- Two medium organic red potatoes with skins on quartered
- Two organic sweet potatoes with skins on quartered
- 8-inch strip kombu
- One bay leaf
- Six black corns
- Three whole allspice or juniper berries
- 1/2 tablespoon sea salt

Directions:
1. Clean the carrots, potatoes, sweet potatoes, and yams well. Rinse the remaining veggies, including the kombu, well. In a large 6-8 quart stockpot, combine all of the ingredients except the salt. Fill the saucepan with water to 2 inches below the rim. Bring to a boil, then reduce to low heat and cook, uncovered, for 2-3 hours. Simmer until the entire richness of the veggies is discernible. Stir in the salt.
2. Strain stock; cool to room temperature before refrigerating or freezing.

Nutrition Facts: Calories: 498 | Carbohydrates: 57 g | Protein: 21 g | Fat: 2 g | Cholesterol: 172 mg

26. CHILE RELLENO CHICKEN SOUP

Prep Time: 15 minutes
Cook Time: 25 minutes
Total Time: 40 minutes
Servings: 8

Ingredients:
- Two tablespoon butter
- Pablano
- 1/4 cup chopped onion
- Two cloves garlic minced
- One tablespoon ground cumin
- 4 cups chicken bone broth
- Salt to taste
- One pound of boneless skinless chicken breast cut into ½ inch pieces
- 8 oz cream cheese cut into cubes
- 3 ½ cups shredded cheddar cheese divided

Directions:
1. Poblano should be roasted until the skin is browned and blistered. You can do this over an open flame on a gas burner or by preheating your broiler too high and setting the poblanos a few inches from the broiler (turning to get all sides charred).
2. Cover with plastic wrap. Allow it cool before rubbing the area to remove as much as possible.
3. Melt the butter in a large saucepan over medium heat. Cook, often turning, until the onion is transparent, about 5 minutes. Stir in the garlic, cumin, and poblanos until fragrant, approximately 1 minute.
4. Stir in the chicken broth and season with salt to taste. Bring to a boil, then reduce to low heat. Cook, occasionally stirring, until the chicken is cooked through, about 10 minutes.
5. Whisk in the cream cheese and two cups of the cheddar cheese until smooth.
6. To serve, divide the mixture into eight bowls and top each with 1/4 cup shredded cheddar cheese. Broil for some minutes, or until the cheese is melted and browned (this step is optional, but OH SO GOOD!).

Nutrition Facts: Calories: 476 | Carbohydrates: 7 g | Protein: 32 g | Fat: 29 g | Cholesterol: 152 mg

27. THAI COCONUT CURRY LENTIL SOUP

Prep Time: 15 minutes
Cook Time: 35 minutes
Total Time: 40 minutes
Servings: 4

Ingredients:
- One tablespoon of olive oil
- One cup of onion finely chopped
- One clove of garlic minced
- One teaspoon ginger minced
- One teaspoon Thai red curry paste use two teaspoons if you like it spicy
- Six cups low sodium vegetable broth
- One cup red lentils picked through for stones, rinsed
- One medium of sweet potato cut into 1/2" pieces
- One stalk lemongrass tender bulb only smashed with a mallet
- Two kaffir lime leaves
- 1/4 teaspoon turmeric
- One teaspoon of sea salt
- 1/4 cup coconut milk

Optional garnish: fresh kaffir lime leaf slivers or chopped cilantro

Directions:
1. In a medium cooking pan, heat the olive oil. Combine the onions, ginger, and garlic in a mixing bowl. Cook for 3-4 minutes over medium heat or until softened.
2. Cook for several minutes or until the Thai red curry paste is aromatic.
3. Combine the broth, lentils, sweet potato, lemongrass, kaffir lime leaves, and turmeric in a mixing bowl. Bring to a boil, then reduce to medium-low heat, cover, and simmer for 20-25 minutes, or until the lentils and sweet potatoes are tender.
4. Remove the lemongrass and kaffir lime leaves from the dish. Stir in the coconut milk and season with salt. Cook for another five minutes. If desired, puree.
5. Garnish with slivers of kaffir lime leaf or fresh cilantro and a drizzle of coconut milk.

Nutrition Facts: Calories: 312 | Carbohydrates: 12 g | Protein: 7 g | Fat: 49 g | Cholesterol: 15 mg

28. LEMON VANILLA BEAN CUSTARD

Prep Time: 10 minutes
Cook Time: 5 minutes
Total Time: 15 minutes
Servings: 4

Ingredients:
- 1 cup (240 ml) canned unsweetened, full-fat coconut milk, stirred before measuring
- ¼ cup (60 ml) honey
- 2 large eggs
- 2 tablespoons fresh lemon juice
- 2 teaspoons fresh lemon zest
- ½ teaspoon vanilla bean paste
- ½ teaspoon pure vanilla extract
- 1 pinch sea salt
- 1 ½ teaspoons powdered gelatin, dissolved in 3 tablespoons boiling water

Directions:
1. In a medium saucepan over low heat, combine the coconut milk, honey, eggs, lemon juice, lemon zest, vanilla bean paste, vanilla essence, and sea salt. Cook, whisking periodically until the coconut milk has melted and the mixture is warm.
2. Cook for 1 minute, frequently whisking, after adding the dissolved gelatin.
3. Pour the custard through a neat sieve into a bowl, cover with plastic wrap, and place in the refrigerator overnight.
4. In a food processor, puree the custard until smooth.

5. Pour the custard into four separate dishes; serve immediately or cover with plastic wrap and refrigerate for up to three days.

Nutrition Facts: Calories: 203 | Carbohydrates: 22 g | Protein: 5 g | Fat: 0 g | Cholesterol: 52 mg

16. When done, the Instant Pot will beep and the screen will display "YOGT." Take off the cover.
17. Place the yogurt in airtight containers.
18. Refrigerate until cool, about 4-6 hours or up to 5 days.

Nutrition Facts: Calories: 104 | Carbohydrates: 9 g | Protein: 7 g | Fat: 10 g | Cholesterol: 251 mg

29. POT KETO YOGURT

Prep Time: 10 minutes
Cook Time: 550 minutes
Total Time: 560 minutes
Servings: 16

Ingredients:
- 4 cups whole milk
- 4 cups heavy cream
- 2 tablespoon plain yogurt

Directions:
1. Fill the Instant Pot halfway with milk and heavy cream.
2. To blend, mix everything together.
3. To choose More mode, continuously press the YOGURT button on the Instant Pot.
4. The Instant Pot will beep after 10 seconds and the screen will say "BOIL."
5. Close the lid and go.
6. When the boil cycle is finished, the LCD will display "YOGT," and the Pot will switch off.
7. Take off the cover.
8. Check the temperature of the milk with a kitchen thermometer.
9. Milk must be heated to at least 180°F.
10. Allow the milk to cool to a temperature of 110 to 115 °F.
11. In a small dish, place 12 cups of milk.
12. Stir in the plain yogurt to mix.
13. Return the yogurt mixture to the saucepan with the milk mixture. Put the cover back on.
14. Adjust to Normal mode by pressing the "Yogurt" button.
15. Set the clock to 8 a.m. Close the box with a lid.

30. BANANA COCONUT CHIA PUDDING

Prep Time: 10 minutes
Cook Time: 10 minutes
Total Time: 20 minutes
Servings: 4

Ingredients:
- 2 cups of full-fat canned of coconut milk (shake, then pour)
- 2 medium of ripe bananas, plus more for serving
- ¼ cup of pure maple syrup
- 1 teaspoon natural vanilla extract
- 3/4 teaspoon ground cinnamon
- Pinch of Celtic sea salt1/4 cup chia
- 2 tablespoons shredded coconut, to serve

Directions:
1. Blend the coconut milk, 1 banana, maple syrup (or another sweetener), vanilla, cinnamon, and salt for 10 to 20 seconds on high until creamy. Whisk in the chia until fully mixed in a glass dish or big jar. Allow standing for about 5 minutes before whisking again.
2. Refrigerate for at least 3 hours or more until thickened.
3. Mash the second banana and fold it into the mixture. Transfer the mixture to 4 serving dishes and top with extra sliced banana and shredded coconut, if desired. If you don't eat it right away, the banana will oxidize.

Nutrition Facts: Calories: 67 | Carbohydrates: 12 g | Protein: 2 g | Fat: 2 g | Cholesterol: 86 mg

31. BANANA PUDDING

Prep Time: 60 minutes
Cook Time: 60 minutes
Total Time: 120 minutes
Servings: 10

Ingredients:
- Three cups heavy whipping cream
- seven egg yolks
- ½ cup of granulated sugar substitute
- 1 ½ teaspoons vanilla extract
- two teaspoons of high-quality banana extract
- two tablespoons of un-salted butter, at room temperature
- 1/8 teaspoon of salt
- 1/8 teaspoon of Xanthan gum to help thicken

Directions:
1. Make a batch of vanilla wafers and then make the pudding while the cookies cool on the baking rack.
2. To create the keto banana pudding, heat the heavy cream in a medium-sized saucepan over low heat until hot.
3. Set aside to cool after adding the vanilla and banana extracts.
4. Whisk the egg yolks and sugar substitute in a medium-sized mixing basin with an electric mixer until the mixture is light yellow.
5. Pour one-quarter of the heavy cream mixture into the egg mixture, xanthan gum, salt, and whisk until fully mixed after the cream has cooled to the touch. The egg yolks will be tempered as a result of this.
6. Once the mixture has been tempered, add the remaining heavy cream, then pour the cream and egg combination back into the saucepan and simmer over low heat for about 7 minutes, or until the mixture begins to thicken, constantly stirring with a wooden spoon. When the pudding is thick enough to coat the back of a wooden spoon without leaking, it's done.
7. Then remove from the fire and whisk in the softened butter until thoroughly blended.
8. Pour the pudding through a fine-mesh sieve into a second medium-sized mixing bowl. To prevent skin from developing, place a sheet of cling wrap immediately over the surface of the pudding.
9. Place the pudding in the refrigerator for at least one hour to chill.

Assemble The Dessert
1. To make the "banana" pudding dessert, place half of the pudding in a trifle dish, followed by 12 biscuits.
2. Next, add another layer of pudding and crumble the remaining 12 cookies on top, or leave them whole and crumble a couple.
3. Refrigerate the dessert for the flavors to combine and the cookies to soften.
4. Refrigerate any leftovers for up to 5 days.

Nutrition Facts: Calories: 230 | Carbohydrates: 2 g | Protein: 2.8 g | Fat: 13 g | Cholesterol: 227 mg

32. CREAM OF MUSHROOM SOUP

Prep Time: 5 minutes
Cook Time: 35 minutes
Total Time: 40 minutes
Servings: 6

Ingredients:
- 4 tablespoons salted butter
- 16 oz mushrooms - sliced
- 1 tablespoon dehydrated minced onion
- 1 tablespoon minced garlic
- 2 cups heavy cream
- 2 cups chicken broth
- ½ teaspoon salt
- ½ teaspoon black
- 1 teaspoon dried thyme
- 4 teaspoons arrowroot
- 8 teaspoons water

Directions:
1. Melt butter in a big saucepan or dutch oven over medium heat.
2. Sauté the onions and garlic for 2-3 minutes, or until aromatic.

3. Sauté the mushrooms for 8-10 minutes, stirring often.
4. Bring the broth to a boil.
5. Return to a boil with the spices and heavy cream. Turn down the heat to low.
6. Make an arrowroot and water slurry (mix them together and stir until smooth).
7. Simmer for 12-15 minutes before adding the arrowroot and stirring. Remove from heat as soon as the sauce thickens.

Nutrition Facts: Calories: 377 | Carbohydrates: 8 g | Protein: 4 g | Fat: 23 g | Cholesterol: 129 mg

33. SUGAR-FREE APPLESAUCE

Prep Time: 10 minutes
Cook Time: 230 minutes
Total Time: 240 minutes
Servings: 12

Ingredients:
- 8 apples peeled and cored. I like to use a combination of Granny Smith and Gala apples.
- ½ tablespoon cinnamon
- ½ cup water
- 2 tablespoon lemon juice

Directions:
Stovetop
1. Apples should be peeled and cored. The apple peeler and corer will expedite the process, but a pairing knife can also be used to cut and core your apples. Reduce the size of the apple chunks.
2. In a stockpot or dutch oven, combine the apples and cinnamon. 12 cup water should be added.
3. Bring the water to a boil. Reduce the heat to low and cover. Cook on low heat for 25-30 minutes. Apples will be broken down but still have a chunky texture.
4. Turn off the heat. Pour in the lemon juice. Mash applesauce with a potato masher or fork for chunky applesauce. Use an immersion blender to make smooth applesauce. Serve hot or cold.

Slow Cooker
1. Apples should be peeled and cored. To speed up the procedure, use an apple peeler and corer or a pairing knife. Cut into smaller pieces.
2. Place the apples in the slow cooker. Garnish with cinnamon. To mix, stir everything together. 12 cups of water should be added.
3. Turn your slow cooker on high and simmer for 4 hours, or until the apples have broken down. Pour in the lemon juice.
4. If your applesauce is chunky, mash it with a potato masher or use an immersion blender to smooth it up. Serve warm or cold.

Instant Pot
1. Apples should be peeled and cut into chunks. To speed up the procedure, use an apple peeler and corer or a paring knife.
2. In the instant pot, combine the cinnamon, lemon, and water. To mix, stir everything together. Mix in the apples. To mix, stir everything together.
3. Place the cover on the instant pot and secure it. Cook for 8 minutes on manual (high heat). Allow the pressure to go naturally.
4. Place in a mixing dish to cool. Pour in the lemon juice. To mix, stir everything together. Applesauce will have a thick texture. For a smoother texture, mash with a potato masher or use an immersion blender. Serve hot or cold.

Nutrition Facts: Calories: 167 | Carbohydrates: 20 g | Protein: 15 g | Fat: 28 g | Cholesterol: 240 mg

34. APPLE ARUGULA FLATBREAD

Prep Time: 15 minutes
Cook Time: 8 minutes
Total Time: 23 minutes
Servings: 4

Ingredients:
Flatbread and Toppings
- 2 apples
- 2 cups arugula
- ¼ cup red onion sliced
- 4 whole wheat or gluten-free flatbreads

Vegan Mozzarella
- ½ cup raw cashews
- 1 cup water
- 3 tablespoon + 2 tablespoon tapioca starch
- 1 tablespoon nutritional yeast
- 1 tablespoon apple cider vinegar
- ½ tablespoon salt
- ¼ tablespoon garlic powder

Directions:
1. Preheat the oven to 350 degrees Fahrenheit.
2. Make the vegan mozzarella by preparing the cashews. 12 cup cashews, soaked overnight. Alternatively, soak cashews in boiling water for 10 minutes. Alternatively, ground the cashews 1/4 cup at a time in a coffee grinder. Select the technique that best fits your time and resources. If you don't have a high-powered blender, I recommend using a coffee grinder.
3. Blend drained and soaked cashews or cashew powder (if using a coffee grinder) with water, tapioca starch, nutritional yeast, apple cider vinegar, salt, and garlic powder in a blender. Blend until the cashews are evenly distributed. It will be quite liquid. This is quite normal.
4. Heat the liquid in a medium skillet over medium heat. Continuously stir. The mixture will start to clump together. Continue to whisk until the mixture thickens and becomes gooey and cheesy. Take the pan off the heat.
5. On four flatbreads, spread vegan mozzarella cheese. 14 cup arugula should be sprinkled on top of each. Apples and red onion thinly sliced Spread equally on top of the arugula on each flatbread. Sprinkle with flakes if desired.
6. Preheat the oven to 350°F for 7 minutes. Broil for an extra minute if you want it crisper.
7. Serve immediately after removing from the oven.

Nutrition Facts: Calories: 73 | Carbohydrates: 7 g | Protein: 1 g | Fat: 0 g | Cholesterol: 52 mg

35. APPLE CHIPS

Prep Time: 10 minutes
Cook Time: 30 minutes
Total Time: 40 minutes
Servings: 6

Ingredients:
Apple Chips
- 6 Granny Smith Apple
- 2 tablespoon cinnamon
- ¼ tablespoon kosher salt

Directions:
1. Using a mandoline, wash and finely slice apples 1/8 of an inch thick. Toss the apple slices with the cinnamon in a large mixing basin.
2. Preheat the air fryer to 300°F. Cook the apples in the air fryer at 300°F for 20 minutes to dry them out. Every 5 minutes, toss and turn the apples to ensure that they cook evenly and that the ones in the center are tossed to the side. Apples will start to shrivel up. If the apples aren't completely dry after 20 minutes, cook in 5-minute increments until all liquid has been eliminated. If the apples appear to be burning, reduce the temperature to 275°F.

3. Crisp the apple chips once they have dried. Increase the temperature to 325°F. Crisp for 6 minutes, tossing the apple chips every 2 minutes.
4. Allow apple chips to cool fully before storing them in an airtight container.

Nutrition Facts: Calories: 96 | Carbohydrates: 26 g | Protein: 1 g | Fat: 1 g | Cholesterol: 27 mg

36. SUGAR-FREE APPLE CRISP

Prep Time: 20 minutes
Cook Time: 25 minutes
Total Time: 45 minutes
Servings: 8

Ingredients:
- 6 Granny Smith Apples organic
- 1 cup apple juice, apple cider or water
- ¼ cup sugar-free cranberries optional
- 2 tablespoon arrowroot powder or corn starch
- 1 tablespoon cinnamon plus ¼ tablespoon for the oats mixture
- ¼ tablespoon ginger
- ½ tablespoon vanilla extract
- 1 tablespoon maple syrup
- 1 cup gluten-free oats
- ¼ cup ground flax
- ¼ cup raw walnuts
- ¼ cup raw pecans
- ¼ tablespoon salt
- ¼ cup maple syrup
- 1 tablespoon almond butter

Directions:
1. Preheat the oven to 350°F.
2. 6 apples, peeled, cored, and sliced
3. Combine sliced apples, cranberries (optional), 1 tablespoon cinnamon, ginger, 1 tablespoon maple syrup, vanilla, arrowroot powder (or corn starch), and apple cider or water.
4. In a mixing bowl, combine oats, ground flax, pecans, walnuts, ¼ cup maple syrup, almond butter, ¼ tablespoon cinnamon, and salt. Pulse until grainy paste forms.
5. Pour the apple mixture into the bottom of a medium baking dish. Over the top, evenly distribute the oat crumble.
6. Bake for 25 minutes, or until the top browns and the apples release their juices and soften.

Nutrition Facts: Calories: 212 | Carbohydrates: 34 g | Protein: 3 g | Fat: 1 g | Cholesterol: 142 mg

37. CHOCOLATE NICE CREAM

Prep Time: 5 minutes
Cook Time: 1 minute
Total Time: 6 minutes
Servings: 4

Ingredients:
- 4 bananas ripened and frozen
- ¼ cup organic cocoa powder
- 1 tablespoon organic vanilla extract
- 1 tablespoon coconut milk or another dairy-free milk (optional)

Directions:
1. Frozen bananas should be cut into pieces. Put everything in a food processor or blender. Blend until the mixture is crumbly.
2. Mix in the chocolate powder and vanilla extract. Blend until everything is properly blended. In the food processor, it will form a ball.
3. If the mixture needs additional liquid to blend effectively, add coconut milk or another dairy-free milk.

Nutrition Facts: Calories: 128 | Carbohydrates: 30 g | Protein: 2 g | Fat: 1 g | Cholesterol: 13 mg

38. HEALTHY WATERMELON POPSICLES

Prep Time: 10 minutes
Cook Time: 180 minutes
Total Time: 190 minutes
Servings: 4

Ingredients:
- 2 cups watermelon cubed
- 1 cup strawberries hulled and halved
- 2 tablespoon vegan chocolate chips or raisins
- ¼ cup coconut milk (full fat) plus 2 tablespoon
- 2 kiwi peeled and cubed

Directions:
1. Watermelon should be cut and cubed. Strawberries should be de-stemmed and sliced into quarters. Blend the 2 cups of watermelon and 1 cup of strawberries in a large mixing bowl until smooth. Fill four popsicle molds about 3/4 full with the mixture.
2. Divide the chocolate chips equally between the four molds. Gently press the chocolate chips into the molds with a popsicle stick, spreading them evenly. Raisins can also be used.
3. Freeze for one hour or until frozen.
4. While the first is frozen, combine 14 cups coconut milk and 1 teaspoon maple syrup. After the initial layer has hardened, equally distribute the coconut milk among the four molds, about 1 tablespoon each mold.
5. Freeze for one further hour or until set.
6. While the second layer is freezing, remove the kiwi's outer covering and slice it into tiny bits. Combine with 2 tablespoons coconut milk.
7. Pour the kiwi layer on top of the coconut layer after it has set. Freeze for another hour or until set. Serve and have fun!

Nutrition Facts: Calories: 174 | Carbohydrates: 26 g | Protein: 3 g | Fat: 9 g | Cholesterol: 356 mg

39. SPINACH MANGO VEGAN POPSICLES

Prep Time: 5 minutes
Cook Time: 180 minutes
Total Time: 185 minutes
Servings: 4

Ingredients:
- 1 cup unsweetened almond milk
- 1 ½ cups fresh spinach
- ⅓ cup unsweetened coconut milk yogurt
- ½ cup frozen mango
- ½ cup frozen banana optional
- 2 tablespoon maple syrup optional

Directions:
1. Blend almond milk and spinach in a blender. Blend on medium-high until the spinach is thoroughly broken down and incorporated.
2. Combine the coconut milk, mango, banana (optional), and maple syrup in a mixing bowl. Blend until completely smooth.
3. Fill Popsicle molds with the mixture. Popsicle sticks should be inserted. If they don't stand straight in the molds, place them in the freezer for an hour before inserting them.
4. For best results, freeze for at least 3 hours, preferably overnight.

Nutrition Facts: Calories: 81 | Carbohydrates: 15 g | Protein: 1 g | Fat: 1 g | Cholesterol: 253 mg

40. MANGO BANANA SMOOTHIE

Prep Time: 5 minutes
Cook Time: 0 minutes
Total Time: 5 minutes
Servings: 2

Ingredients:
- 1 cup frozen cubed mango
- 1 frozen banana chopped
- 1 cup unsweetened almond milk

- ¼ cup dairy-free coconut milk yogurt plain unsweetened
- 1 scoop pea protein powder optional

Directions:
1. Fill your blender or smoothie cup with almond milk, coconut yogurt, protein powder, fresh mangoes, and chopped frozen banana in the following order: almond milk, coconut yogurt, protein powder, fresh mangoes, and chopped frozen banana.
2. Connect the blender lid or the smoothie attachment blade. Begin on low and gradually increase speed until all items are thoroughly mixed.
3. Pour the mixture into two glasses. Serve with fresh mango, chia, and coconut flakes on top (optional)

Nutrition Facts: Calories: 193 | Carbohydrates: 30 g | Protein: 14 g | Fat: 1 g | Cholesterol: 318 mg

41. SPINACH BLUEBERRY SMOOTHIE

Prep Time: 3 minutes
Cook Time: 2 minutes
Total Time: 5 minutes
Servings: 1

Ingredients:
- 1 cup almond milk unsweetened vanilla or regular
- 1 cup raw spinach loosely packed
- 1 frozen banana chopped into chunks
- ½ cup frozen blueberries
- 1 tablespoon chia

Directions:
1. In a blender, combine the ingredients in the sequence listed in the recipe, beginning with the almond milk and working your way up to the spinach, frozen banana, frozen blueberries, and chia. Blend until completely smooth.

Nutrition Facts: Calories: 247 | Carbohydrates: 45 g | Protein: 6 g | Fat: 1 g | Cholesterol: 261 mg

42. SNOWMAN CHRISTMAS SMOOTHIE

Prep Time: 5 minutes
Cook Time: 0 minutes
Total Time: 5 minutes
Servings: 2

Ingredients:
- 1 banana frozen and chopped
- 1 cup unsweetened almond milk
- ¼ cup desiccated coconut shredded, unsweetened
- ½ cup coconut whipped cream optional
- blue sugar sprinkles optional

Directions:
1. Assemble the Snowman cups. To construct the mouth, draw two circular eyes, one triangular nose, and 5-6 tiny circles in a curved shape.
2. In a blender, combine the almond milk, banana, and coconut.
3. Blend until completely smooth. Approximately 5-10 seconds
4. Pour the smoothie into the glasses. Sprinkle with blue sugar sprinkles and top with coconut whipped cream.

Nutrition Facts: Calories: 51 | Carbohydrates: 17 g | Protein: 8 g | Fat: 6 g | Cholesterol: 201 mg

43. CLEAN GREEN SHAMROCK SHAKE

Prep Time: 5 minutes
Cook Time: 0 minutes
Total Time: 5 minutes
Servings: 1

Ingredients:

- 1 cup light Coconut Milk
- ¼ avocado
- 1 banana frozen
- ½ cup fresh leaf spinach
- ⅛ tablespoon peppermint extract
- 1 tablespoon dairy-free chocolate chips optional

Directions:
1. In a blender, combine the frozen banana, coconut milk, avocado, spinach, and peppermint essence. Blend until smooth and well blended.
2. Fill a glass halfway with ice and top with chocolate chunks.

Nutrition Facts: Calories: 382 | Carbohydrates: 41 g | Protein: 3 g | Fat: 23 g | Cholesterol: 183 mg

44. PUMPKIN SMOOTHIE

Prep Time: 3 minutes
Cook Time: 0 minutes
Total Time: 3 minutes
Servings: 2

Ingredients:
- 1 banana frozen
- ½ cup pumpkin puree
- 1 cup almond milk unsweetened
- ½ tablespoon pumpkin pie spice
- 1 tablespoon maple syrup optional
- ½ cup ice cubes

Directions:
1. In a blender, combine the frozen banana, pumpkin purée, almond milk, pumpkin pie spice, and maple syrup.
2. Blend until the mixture is smooth and creamy. If using a high-speed blender, start at the lowest level and gradually increase to 5 or 6 until all components are incorporated. Blend in the ice until well mixed.
3. Pour the mixture into two glasses. Serve with a sprinkling of pumpkin pie spice on top.

Nutrition Facts: Calories: 119 | Carbohydrates: 26 g | Protein: 2 g | Fat: 1 g | Cholesterol: 19 mg

45. PROTEIN BALLS WITH PEANUT BUTTER AND CHOCOLATE CHIPS

Prep Time: 15 minutes
Cook Time: 0 minutes
Total Time: 15 minutes
Servings: 16

Ingredients:
- ½ cup Natural Organic Peanut Butter
- ½ cup Ground Flax
- 1 cup Organic Oats Bob's Red Mill is Gluten Free
- 2 tablespoon Organic Maple Syrup
- ¼ cup Organic Semi-Sweet Chocolate Chips

Directions:
1. Combine the peanut butter, flax, oats, and maple syrup in a mixing bowl. Stir until everything is well combined. The consistency will be a little dry.
2. Add the chocolate chips and mix well.
3. Scoop a spoonful of the mixture and roll into balls with a small tablespoon (ice cream) scoop. Continue until the entire mixture has been used. Allow for an hour of chilling before serving.

Nutrition Facts: Calories: 114 | Carbohydrates: 10 g | Protein: 4 g | Fat: 2 g | Cholesterol: 41 mg

46. COOKIE DOUGH BALLS

Prep Time: 5 minutes
Cook Time: 30 minutes
Total Time: 35 minutes
Servings: 18

Ingredients:
- 1 cup almond flour blanched

- 2 tablespoon maple syrup
- 3 tablespoon almond butter
- 1 tablespoon vanilla extract
- 3 tablespoon chocolate chips

Directions:
1. Fill a mixing bowl halfway with almond flour. Pour in the maple syrup, almond butter, and vanilla extract.
2. Stir until everything is fully mixed. It will have a crumbly feel but will hold together when rolled into balls.
3. Stir in the chocolate chunks.
4. 1 tablespoon of dough, rolled into a ball Rep with the remaining balls.
5. Refrigerate in an airtight container for 30 minutes to harden and set.

Nutrition Facts: Calories: 59 | Carbohydrates: 3 g | Protein: 2 g | Fat: 1 g | Cholesterol: 29 mg

47. GLUTEN-FREE PUMPKIN PIE BARS

Prep Time: 15 minutes
Cook Time: 80 minutes
Total Time: 95 minutes
Servings: 9

Ingredients:
- 1 cup gluten-free oats
- 1 cup blanched almond flour
- ¼ cup raw almond butter
- ¼ cup ground flax
- 3 tablespoon organic maple syrup
- ¼ tablespoon salt
- 3 cups pumpkin puree
- ¼ cup coconut milk full fat in can
- ¼ cup maple syrup
- ¼ cup date sugar
- 2 tablespoon arrowroot powder
- 2 tablespoon pumpkin pie spice
- ½ tablespoon salt

Directions:
1. Preheat the oven to 350 degrees Fahrenheit.
2. In a food processor, combine oats, almond flour, flax, almond butter, maple syrup, and salt. Pulse until the mixture is crumbly.
3. Line an 8-by-8-inch square baking pan with parchment paper. Evenly press the crust into the pan. Bake for 20 minutes at 350°F.
4. While the crust is baking, in a food processor, mix the pumpkin puree, coconut milk, maple syrup, arrowroot powder, pumpkin pie spice, and salt. To mix, pulse many times.
5. Allow the crust to cool after it has been removed from the oven. Then, on top, add the pumpkin pie filling. Distribute evenly. To level out the filling and eliminate any bubbles, lightly tap the pan on the counter.
6. Bake for 50-60 minutes at 350°F. When the pie comes out of the oven, it must be totally cool. Allow the pie to cool completely at room temperature before covering and transferring to the refrigerator to set for at least 4 hours. Allow sitting overnight if cooking this pie ahead of time. The longer you let the pie set, the less watery it will be. Overnight is the greatest option.
7. When the pie has completely cooled, gently lift the parchment paper ends to release the pie from the pan. Cut the ends of each side with a sharp knife to create a clean finish. Measure 2.5 inches across the big square's left side and bottom. Gently use a knife to measure across and over the top of the huge square to create a grid, then firmly push your knife on the lines to cut 9 equal squares.

Nutrition Facts: Calories: 211 | Carbohydrates: 28 g | Protein: 61 g | Fat: 2 g | Cholesterol: 172 mg

48. HEALTHY VEGAN BROWNIES

Prep Time: 15 minutes
Cook Time: 30 minutes
Total Time: 45 minutes

Servings: 9

Ingredients:
- 4 tablespoon ground flax
- ⅔ cup warm water
- 1 cup date sugar or coconut sugar
- 1 cup cacao powder
- ½ cup white whole wheat flour
- ½ tablespoon salt
- 1 tablespoon baking powder
- ½ cup unsweetened applesauce or pumpkin puree
- 1 tablespoon vanilla extract
- ¼ cup unsweetened almond milk optional

Directions:
1. Preheat the oven to 325 degrees Fahrenheit. In a small dish, combine ground flax and warm water. Allow for a 15-minute resting period.
2. In a medium mixing bowl, combine the dry ingredients (date sugar, cacao powder, white whole wheat flour, baking powder, and salt) while the flax egg is setting.
3. In the middle of the dry ingredients, make a well. Combine the wet and dry components (flax egg, applesauce/or pumpkin puree, and vanilla extract). Stir until well mixed. If the batter appears to be too dry, add 14 cups of unsweetened almond milk.
4. Pour the batter into an 8-inch square baking dish lined with parchment paper. Distribute evenly.
5. Bake for 30-35 minutes, or until a toothpick inserted into the center comes out clean. Allow cooling fully in the pan before removing and cutting into squares.

Nutrition Facts: Calories: 126 | Carbohydrates: 28 g | Protein: 3 g | Fat: 1 g | Cholesterol: 172 mg

49. CHOCOLATE CHIA PUDDING

Prep Time: 5 minutes
Cook Time: 5 minutes
Total Time: 10 minutes
Servings: 4

Ingredients:
- ¼ cup chia
- 2 tablespoon granulated Stevia or another low carb sweetener to taste
- 2 tablespoon unsweetened cocoa powder
- 1 tablespoon vanilla extract
- 1 cup unsweetened almond milk

Directions:
1. Combine the chia, cocoa powder, and sweetener in a mixing dish.
2. Combine the almond milk and vanilla essence in a mixing bowl.
3. Refrigerate overnight, wrapped with plastic wrap.
4. Serve with your preferred fruit.

Nutrition Facts: Calories: 82 | Carbohydrates: 8 g | Protein: 3 g | Fat: 5 g | Cholesterol: 91 mg

50. GREEN SMOOTHIE RECIPE

Prep Time: 2 minutes
Cook Time: 3 minutes
Total Time: 5 minutes
Servings: 2

Ingredients:
- 1 cup fresh spinach
- 1 cup water
- 1/2 cup pineapple, frozen
- 1/2 cup mango, frozen
- 1 banana
- 1 Protein Smoothie Boost, optional

Directions:
1. Measure Fill a measuring cup halfway with spinach.
2. Add Blend the spinach with the water in a blender. Blend until all of the chunks are gone. (When thoroughly mixed, the mixture should resemble green water.)

3. In a blender, combine the pineapple, mango, and banana. To save time chopping and preparing, I use frozen pineapple and mangos to cool the smoothie. It's a win-win situation!
4. Blend everything until smooth and creamy. This might take as short as 30 seconds or as long as 2 minutes, depending on your blender.
5. Pour into a glass and serve right away.
6. Refrigerate with a cover in the fridge until ready to consume.

Nutrition Facts: Calories: 203 | Carbohydrates: 51 g | Protein: 3 g | Fat: 1 g | Cholesterol: 88 mg

51. KEY LIME MOUSSE

Prep Time: 10 minutes
Cook Time: 60 minutes
Total Time: 70 minutes
Servings: 8

Ingredients:
- 1 envelope grass-fed gelatin about 7 grams or 2 ½ teaspoons
- ¼ cup cold water
- ⅓ cup boiling water
- ½ cup low carb sugar substitute or more to taste (see note)
- 1 tablespoon lime zest
- 2 cups cold whipping cream
- ⅔ cup key lime juice

Directions:
1. In a small dish, sprinkle gelatin over cold water and let it aside for 2 minutes to soften. Stir in the boiling water until the gelatin is completely dissolved and the liquid is clear. Allow cooling slightly.
2. In a large mixing bowl, combine the sweetener and lime zest. Whip the cream with an electric mixer until firm peaks form.
3. Pour in the gelatin mixture as well as the key lime juice. Continue to beat until everything is properly combined.
4. Refrigerate for at least two hours or until the mousse is firm. Refrigerate covered in the refrigerator.

Nutrition Facts: Calories: 309 | Carbohydrates: 2 g | Protein: 25 g | Fat: 14 g | Cholesterol: 80 mg

52. FUDGY SWEET POTATO BROWNIES

Prep Time: 10 minutes
Cook Time: 28 minutes
Total Time: 38 minutes
Servings: 8

Ingredients:
- 1 cup mashed sweet potato
- ¼ cup maple syrup
- ¼ cup almond butter
- ¼ cup coconut oil, melted
- 1 teaspoon vanilla
- ½ cup cocoa powder
- ¼ cup coconut flour
- Pinch sea salt
- ½ cup dairy-free chocolate chips (~50 grams)

Directions:
1. Preheat the oven to 350 degrees Fahrenheit and line a loaf pan with parchment paper.
2. In a large mixing bowl, combine the sweet potato, maple syrup, almond butter, coconut oil, and vanilla extract until smooth.
3. After that, stir in the cocoa powder, coconut flour, and sea salt until a smooth batter forms.
4. Combine the chocolate chips using a spatula.
5. Pour the batter into the prepared loaf pan and push it down until level.
6. Cook for 25-28 minutes, or until a knife inserted into the middle comes out clean.

7. Allow the brownies to cool in the loaf pan before carefully removing them from the pan and cutting them into squares with the parchment paper.
8. Any leftovers can be stored in an airtight container for up to a few days.

Nutrition Facts: Calories: 274 | Carbohydrates: 0 g | Protein: 16 g | Fat: 18 g | Cholesterol: 86 mg

53. BREAKFAST SMOOTHIE

Prep Time: 5 minutes
Cook Time: 3 minutes
Total Time: 8 minutes
Servings: 2

Ingredients:
- 2 bananas
- 15 oz can peaches, undrained, or 2 cups fresh sliced peaches
- 1 1/2 cups fresh or frozen raspberries, blueberries and blackberries (I use frozen berries for a thicker smoothie but you can always add ice)
- 1/2 cup old-fashioned rolled oats
- 1 cup plain Greek yogurt or your favorite flavor
- large handful ice

Directions:
1. Fill your blender halfway with fresh or frozen fruit. Pour in the liquid (milk, water, or low-sugar fruit juice). Combine old-fashioned oats, Greek yogurt, and a handful of ice in a mixing bowl.
2. Blend until completely smooth. Add more ice (to thicken) or liquid (to thin) until the desired consistency is reached.

Nutrition Facts: Calories: 192 | Carbohydrates: 39 g | Protein: 8 g | Fat: 1 g | Cholesterol: 251 mg

54. POTATO LEEK SOUP

Prep Time: 10 minutes
Cook Time: 20 minutes
Total Time: 30 minutes
Servings: 4

Ingredients:
- 1 teaspoon olive oil, optional
- 2 large leeks, washed and sliced thinly (use just the white and light green parts)
- 1125g | 5 cups potato, peeled and cubed
- 960mls | 4 cups water
- 1 can (398-400mls / 13.5 oz) light coconut milk; it must be light if you don't want to taste coconut in the finished soup *
- 1/4 teaspoon ground nutmeg
- 2 teaspoons salt
- 4-5 sprigs of fresh thyme or 1/4 teaspoon of dried thyme (optional)

Optional Croutons
- Cubed bread Gluten-free if necessary, and it's better if it's a few days old
- Olive oil
- Salt

Directions:
1. In a soup pot, heat the oil over medium heat. If you want to cook without oil, sauté them in a few tablespoons of water and add a little more as needed to prevent sticking.
2. Sauté the sliced leeks for 5 minutes, or until they begin to color.
3. Cook for another minute or two after adding the potato.
4. Simmer, covered with water, until the potato is soft (test with a fork - it will take about 10 minutes).
5. Take the pan off the heat and stir in the spice, coconut milk, and nutmeg.
6. Remove the thyme leaves from the stems with your fingers and add them to the soup.
7. Blend in a blender or with an immersion blender until smooth and creamy.
8. Return to the pan and reheat through on medium-low heat before serving.
9. Croutons are optional.
10. Preheat the oven to 300°F.
11. Stir bread cubes in a basin with olive oil or sprinkle with oil and toss thoroughly.

12. Sprinkle with salt before pouring onto a baking pan and spreading out into a single layer.
13. Place in the oven and bake until dry and golden brown. Keep an eye on them because they don't take long. (5–10 minutes, with a maximum of 15 minutes).
14. Cool and store in an airtight jar.

Nutrition Facts: Calories: 299 | Carbohydrates: 54 g | Protein: 6 g | Fat: 7 g | Cholesterol: 231 mg

55. TOMATO PASTA BAKE WITH GARLICKY CRUMB TOPPING

Prep Time: 20 minutes
Cook Time: 30 minutes
Total Time: 50 minutes
Servings: 5

Ingredients:
For the pasta
- 500 g pasta uses gluten-free pasta to make gluten-free; fusilli or rigatoni both work well.
- 1 tablespoon olive oil to make oil-free; just use a few drops of water instead
- 1 large onion
- 3 fat cloves of garlic
- 1 large can | 28fl oz/ 796mls crushed tomatoes You can sub this for passata or blend up a can of diced tomatoes until smooth if that is all you have
- ½ teaspoon chili flakes
- 2 teaspoons mixed Italian dried herbs feel free to sub for any dried herbs you like
- ¼ cup | 4 tablespoons nutritional yeast adds depth of flavor to the sauce - DO NOT sub for any other type of yeast
- 1 tablespoon balsamic vinegar
- 1 teaspoon salt
- ½ teaspoon ground black

For the topping
- 5 medium cut slices slightly stale bread | You can use a bit more if you have lots to use up or you can use a bit less | Use gluten-free bread to keep the recipe gluten-free
- 2 tablespoons olive oil optional but recommended
- 2 cloves garlic
- 2 tablespoons nutritional yeast

Directions:
1. Preheat the oven to 400 degrees Fahrenheit.
2. In a saucepan, heat the olive oil and sauté the onions until they are golden brown. If you don't want to use any oil, use a few drops of water for the olive oil.
3. Cook for another minute after adding the garlic.
4. Stir in the tomatoes, chiles, herbs, nutritional yeast, balsamic vinegar, salt. Allow boiling on low heat while you prepare the pasta.
5. Cook pasta till al dente in a large pot of boiling water.
6. While the pasta is cooking, coarsely break up the bread with your hands and place it in the bowl of a food processor or blender. Combine 2 tablespoons olive oil, garlic, and nutritional yeast in a mixing bowl. Process until the mixture resembles fine crumbs. Place aside.
7. After draining the pasta, add the sauce and mix well to incorporate.
8. Pour the saucy pasta into a large casserole dish, level the top with a spoon, and then equally sprinkle with the breadcrumb mixture.
9. Bake for 20–25 minutes, or until the crumbs are brown and crispy.

Nutrition Facts: Calories: 470 | Carbohydrates: 80 g | Protein: 17 g | Fat: 9 g | Cholesterol: 26 mg

56. CREAMY CAULIFLOWER HORSERADISH SOUP

Prep Time: 5 minutes
Cook Time: 15 minutes
Total Time: 20 minutes
Servings: 4

Ingredients:

- 1 medium cauliflower broken or chopped into pieces (stalks as well)
- 2 medium potatoes chopped, chopped
- 1 medium onion, chopped roughly
- 2 cloves garlic, chopped
- 720mls | 3 cups vegetable broth
- 1 teaspoon dried thyme
- 240mls | 1 cup non-dairy milk (any kind as long as it is unsweetened)
- 2 - 4 teaspoons horseradish sauce (add to taste)
- salt

Directions:

1. In a large saucepan, combine the onion, potatoes, cauliflower, garlic, vegetable broth, milk, and thyme.
2. Bring to a boil, then reduce to a simmer, and cook until the potatoes and cauliflower are cooked (check with a fork or knife - it will take about 15 mins max).
3. Blend until fully smooth in a blender or with a stick blender.
4. Return the pan to the heat and season with horseradish to taste. The amount you'll need is determined by how spicy the horseradish is and how pungent you want your soup to be. Continue to taste as you go until it's correct for you.
5. Season to taste with salt.

Nutrition Facts: Calories: 160 | Carbohydrates: 31 g | Protein: 6 g | Fat: 2 g | Cholesterol: 130 mg

57. CARROT SOUP

Prep Time: 10 minutes
Cook Time: 50 minutes
Total Time: 60 minutes
Servings: 8

Ingredients:

- 10 large carrots
- 1 medium onion
- 3-4 inch long fresh ginger root
- 1 tablespoon oil (coconut oil or any other mild tasting oil suitable for roasting) - see recipe notes for an oil-free option
- 400mls / 1 can coconut milk
- 960mls / 4 cups water (around 1000 MLS)
- salt

Directions:

1. Preheat the oven to 400 degrees Fahrenheit.
2. Carrots should be peeled. Cut into big bits (approximately one-inch length).
3. Peel and cut the onion into roughly the same size bits as the carrot.
4. Cut the ginger into two or three pieces. Don't be concerned about peeling it.
5. Cook until the veggies (including the ginger) are soft in a small ovenproof pan coated with oil. It took me approximately 50 minutes to do mine. Prod them with a fork to see whether they're ready.
6. Take the veggies out of the oven.
7. In a blender, combine the veggies and liquid.
8. You'll most likely need to perform this in two or three batches. In the first batch, use coconut milk; in future batches, use water. Just enough for the veggies to be pureed.
9. Once everything is smooth and creamy, pour it into a pan, add any residual water, and season with salt to taste. I used 3 teaspoons salt, but everyone's tastes differ, so use as much or as little as you need.
10. Warm gently in the pan before serving.

Nutrition Facts: Calories: 144 | Carbohydrates: 12 g | Protein: 1 g | Fat: 2 g | Cholesterol: 80 mg

58. STRAWBERRY OVERNIGHT OATS

Prep Time: 5 minutes
Cook Time: 0 minutes
Total Time: 5 minutes
Servings: 1

Ingredients:
- ½ cup (50 grams) rolled or old-fashioned oats, use certified gluten-free oats if necessary
- 1 tablespoon chia
- ¾ cup (180 ml) non-dairy milk
- ½ teaspoon vanilla extract
- 1 tablespoon maple syrup (OPTIONAL), use real maple syrup, not pancake syrup
- 1 tablespoon strawberry jam (OPTIONAL - but recommended)
- Around ½ cup (60 grams) fresh strawberries, chopped

Directions:
1. Add the oats and chia to a jar (or another covered container).
2. Stir in the milk, vanilla extract, and optional maple syrup.
3. Pour in the strawberry jam, followed by the cut strawberries.
4. Place the container in the fridge for at least 3 to 4 hours, but up to 72 hours is OK.
5. Eat the oats straight from the jar, or transfer them to a bowl beforehand.

Nutrition Facts: Calories: 388 | Carbohydrates: 61 g | Protein: 14 g | Fat: 10 g | Cholesterol: 386 mg

59. GINGER PEACH SMOOTHIE

Prep Time: 5 minutes
Cook Time: 5 minutes
Total Time: 10 minutes
Servings: 1

Ingredients:
- 2 ripe, juicy peaches, (You can use frozen peaches, but if you do, use a fresh banana and not a frozen one)
- 1 medium frozen banana (fresh or frozen)
- ¾ cup (180 MLS) non-dairy milk
- 1 tablespoon maple syrup (optional - add to taste or not at all)
- 1 approx 2½ inches long stick fresh ginger, roughly x ½inch wide
- OR ¼ to ½ teaspoon ground ginger

Directions:
1. Remove the pits from the peaches and combine them with the remaining ingredients in a blender. I recommend using only half of the fresh ginger or 14 teaspoons of ground ginger to begin.
2. Blend until smooth, then taste it. If you want a stronger flavor, add a little more ginger.
3. Serve right away.

Nutrition Facts: Calories: 337 | Carbohydrates: 72 g | Protein: 9 g | Fat: 4 g | Cholesterol: 186 mg

60. STRAWBERRY BANANA PEANUT BUTTER SMOOTHIE

Prep Time: 5 minutes
Cook Time: 5 minutes
Total Time: 10 minutes
Servings: 1

Ingredients:
- 2 cups (approx 288 grams) strawberries, fresh or frozen
- 1 medium frozen banana, fresh and not frozen if using frozen strawberries
- 2 tablespoons peanut butter, or any other nut or butter
- 1 cup (240 ml) plant milk, of choice

Optional
- 1 tablespoon maple syrup, or a Medjool date
- 1 tablespoon flax
- 1 tablespoon chia

Directions:

1. In a blender, combine all of the ingredients.
2. Blend until completely smooth.
3. Check the sweetness and, if required, add the optional maple syrup or date, then mix again to combine.

Nutrition Facts: Calories: 465 | Carbohydrates: 60 g | Protein: 18 g | Fat: 21 g | Cholesterol: 276 mg

61. GRANOLA

Prep Time: 5 minutes
Cook Time: 20 minutes
Total Time: 25 minutes
Servings: 6

Ingredients:
- 2 cups (180 grams) rolled or old fashioned oats, use certified gluten-free for gluten-free granola
- 1 cup (85 grams) raw almonds of choice, pecans, walnuts, etc. (or more pumpkin or sunflower for nut-free)
- ½ cup (80 grams) shelled pumpkin, sunflower or hemp, or a mix of all 3
- ½ cup (25 grams) puffed rice (optional) (adds fantastic texture - If you don't use it, make up the quantity with more oats.)
- 6 tablespoons creamy butter of choice
- ¾ cup (180 ml) brown rice syrup or maple syrup, brown rice syrup will give you bigger clusters
- ½ teaspoon fine sea salt, note that if you use iodized (table) salt instead, you will need to use less
- 1 teaspoon ground cinnamon
- 1 teaspoon vanilla extract
- 1 cup dried raisins, sultanas, cranberries, tart cherries or chocolate chips, or any other dried fruit (chopped if it's something like apricots or dates)

Directions:
1. Preheat the oven to 350°F (175°C) and place a shelf on the bottom level.
2. Using parchment paper or a silicone baking mat, line a large baking pan.
3. Add the oats and optional puffed rice to a large mixing bowl. To mix, stir everything together.
4. In a medium mixing bowl, combine the butter, syrup, salt, cinnamon, and vanilla extract. To mix, whisk everything together.
5. Pour the wet mixture into the oaty mixture and stir with a wooden spoon or spatula until everything is mixed, moist, and sticky.
6. Spread it evenly over the prepared tray, about 3/4 inch deep.
7. Bake for 10 minutes on the lowest oven shelf, then take from the oven and stir with a spatula to ensure equal cooking. After you've finished swirling it, firmly press it all over with a spatula or the bottom of a cup. This helps it cling together and forms wonderful large clumps when crumbled later.
8. Return to the oven and bake for another 10 to 15 minutes, or until the top is brown and the house smells toasty.
9. Remove from the oven and sprinkle with the dried fruit/chocolate chips, then leave to cool fully on the baking tray. As it cools, the granola will solidify.
10. Break up the granola into chunky pieces with your hands and place it in an airtight container. It will last 6 to 8 weeks.

Nutrition Facts: Calories: 250 | Carbohydrates: 35 g | Protein: 8 g | Fat: 13 g | Cholesterol: 621 mg

62. PERSIMMON SMOOTHIE

Prep Time: 5 minutes
Cook Time: 5 minutes
Total Time: 10 minutes
Servings: 1

Ingredients:
- 2 medium ripe persimmon
- 1 medium frozen banana
- 1 cup dairy-free milk

- About 10 cashews; if you don't have a high-powered blender, soak the cashew in hot water for 5 minutes before adding to the blender. See notes for cashew alternatives.
- ¼ teaspoon cinnamon, add a little more if you prefer a stronger cinnamon taste
- 1 tablespoon maple syrup

Directions:
1. Remove and discard the persimmon leaves, then chop each fruit into a few pieces. Blend them, together with the remaining ingredients except for the maple syrup, in a blender until smooth.
2. Use the blender to give it a brief taste and, if required, add the maple syrup. After adding it, give it a brisk 5-second mix before serving.

Nutrition Facts: Calories: 298 | Carbohydrates: 41 g | Protein: 11 g | Fat: 12 g | Cholesterol: 121 mg

63. CRANBERRY SMOOTHIE

Prep Time: 5 minutes
Cook Time: 0 minutes
Total Time: 5 minutes
Servings: 1

Ingredients:
- 75g / ¾ cup frozen cranberries (or fresh cranberries but add a handful of ice too)
- 1 large apple cored and chopped into chunks
- 1 small handful / about 2 tablespoons raw pecans or walnuts (see notes for nut-free option)
- 1 tablespoon maple syrup
- 240mls / 1 cup non-dairy milk
- ¼ teaspoon ground cinnamon

Directions:
1. Add all the ingredients to a blender.
2. Blend until smooth.

Nutrition Facts: Calories: 424 | Carbohydrates: 61 g | Protein: 10 g | Fat: 19 g | Cholesterol: 251 mg

64. KALE APPLE SMOOTHIE

Prep Time: 5 minutes
Cook Time: 5 minutes
Total Time: 10 minutes
Servings: 1

Ingredients:
- 2 large kale leaves, washed with stems removed. Use a couple of handfuls of baby kale instead for a milder kale flavor
- 1 large apple, cored (no need to peel unless you want to).
- 1 tablespoon chia
- 2 teaspoons ground flax or whole flax
- 1 - 2 tablespoons maple syrup
- ½ medium lemon, juice only
- 180mls / ¾ cup plant-based milk, add up to a ¼ cup more to thin if you prefer it that way
- 5 ice cubes, OPTIONAL but will make it colder and a bit thicker
- 1 tablespoon almond butter, OPTIONAL - It's great with or without

Directions:
1. Blend all of the ingredients in a blender until smooth. On my Blendtec, I use the smoothie option.
2. Check the sweetness and, if required, add a bit more maple syrup.
3. Serve right away.

Nutrition Facts: Calories: 319 | Carbohydrates: 63 g | Protein: 9 g | Fat: 7 g | Cholesterol: 266 mg

65. GLOWING SKIN SMOOTHIE

Prep Time: 5 minutes
Cook Time: 5 minutes
Total Time: 10 minutes
Servings: 2

Ingredients:
- ¼ cup cashew pieces or 1 very heaping ¼ cup of whole ones about 38g

- 1 cup | 240mls water or coconut water for an extra skin boost!
- 1 medium banana
- 1 very heaping cup frozen mango pieces around 140g, see recipe notes if you only have fresh mango
- 1 tablespoon chia, optional
- ⅛ teaspoon vanilla bean powder or ½ teaspoon vanilla extract
- ½ teaspoon ground cardamon
- ¼ teaspoon ground turmeric
- ⅛ teaspoon ground ginger or a small piece of fresh ginger
- 1 tablespoon of maple syrup or 1 large Medjool date

Directions:
1. If you don't have a high-powered blender, soak the cashew in boiling water for 15 minutes or cold water for 2 hours (this technique will maintain the nutrients), then drain.
2. Blend the cashew with the water in a blender until smooth. You've just created cashew milk!
3. Add the other ingredients and mix until smooth.
4. Serve with a decorative sprinkling of cardamon and turmeric if desired.

Nutrition Facts: Calories: 342 | Carbohydrates: 70 g | Protein: 8 g | Fat: 15 g | Cholesterol: 82 mg

66. CRANBERRY SAUCE

Prep Time: 5 minutes
Cook Time: 15 minutes
Total Time: 20 minutes
Servings: 16

Ingredients:
- 24 oz / 680 g fresh or frozen cranberries
- ½ cup / 100 g sugar, granulated white or cane sugar is best
- ½ cup / 120 ml maple syrup (real, natural maple syrup, not pancake syrup)
- ⅓ cup / 80 mls vegan red wine or port, or orange juice for an alcohol-free alternative
- 1 large orange, zest and juice of
- 1 medium cinnamon stick
- 1 approx 3-inch piece of fresh rosemary

Directions:
To make on the stovetop
1. Wash the cranberries and remove any that are soft. 1 cup of them should be set aside, and the rest should be combined with everything else in a medium saucepan. Cook, frequently stirring, over medium heat until the sauce thickens and becomes jammy and the cranberries break down. Usually, it takes approximately 15 minutes.
2. Remove the rosemary and cinnamon stick from the pan and set aside. Take a quick taste, but be careful because it will be extremely hot. If you want to add more sugar, do so now because it will dissolve in the heat. But keep in mind that it's intended to taste tart. Its purpose is to cut through the richness of your holiday fare.
3. Stir in the cranberries that have been set aside. The residual heat will cook them sufficiently before the sauce cools, giving them a good texture.
4. Allow cooling completely before transferring to sterilized jars or freezer-safe containers.

To make in an Instant Pot
1. Wash the cranberries and remove any that are soft. Scoop out approximately 1 cup and set aside till the end. Place the remaining ingredients in the Instant Pot.
2. Stir in the sugar, maple syrup, red wine, orange juice, and zest. On top, place the cinnamon stick and rosemary.
3. Close the vent and replace the cover on the Instant Pot. Cook for 3 minutes on high pressure before allowing the pressure to naturally release. Open the lid once the pin has dropped. Don't be alarmed if it appears frothy and unappealing. Remove the cinnamon stick and rosemary, and then stir in the saved cranberries.

4. The remaining heat is sufficient to cook them. Stir everything together thoroughly. It now appears to be in good condition. Take a short sip. Take cautious since it will be quite hot. If you find it too sour, add a bit of extra sugar now since it will dissolve in the heat. But keep in mind that a little acidity is excellent since it pairs well with your rich holiday meals.
5. Allow cooling completely before using. At this stage, the lid can be on or off, although it will cool faster with the cover off. Decant into jars or freezer-safe containers once cold.

Nutrition Facts: Calories: 74 | Carbohydrates: 18 g | Protein: 1 g | Fat: 1 g | Cholesterol: 80 mg

67. CHOCOLATE TAHINI PUMPKIN SMOOTHIE

Prep Time: 5 minutes
Cook Time: 0 minutes
Total Time: 5 minutes
Servings: 1

Ingredients:
- 1 frozen banana
- 1 tablespoon cocoa
- 8 tablespoons | ½ cup pumpkin puree canned or fresh
- 1 slightly heaping tablespoon tahini
- 2 tablespoons maple syrup
- 180mls | ¾ cup non-dairy milk

Directions:
1. Add all ingredients to a blender.
2. Blend until completely smooth.
3. Serve immediately.

Nutrition Facts: Calories: 383 | Carbohydrates: 73 g | Protein: 7 g | Fat: 11 g | Cholesterol: 32 mg

68. CARAMEL SAUCE

Prep Time: 2 minutes
Cook Time: 3 minutes
Total Time: 5 minutes
Servings: 4

Ingredients:
- 100g | 1/2 cup coconut sugar (sometimes called coconut palm sugar (I have not tried this with any other sugar, so I can't guarantee it will work as well if you make a sub)
- 2 tablespoons water
- 2 tablespoons tahini (see recipe note)
- 2 tablespoons vegan butter or coconut oil (solid measurement)
- 1/8 - 1/4 teaspoon salt (add to taste)

Directions:
1. In a saucepan, combine the coconut sugar and water.
2. Cook over medium heat until the sugar has fully dissolved and the mixture is just beginning to bubble. DON'T STIR!! Swirl the pan a little if necessary. It will take no more than two to three minutes. If you leave it unattended for too long, it will quickly burn.
3. Take the pan off the heat and stir in the tahini, salt, and vegan butter or coconut oil. Stir vigorously until everything is fully incorporated. It's natural to see a few bright specks through it. If you're having problems getting it to come together, place it back over low heat for 30 seconds or so.

Nutrition Facts: Calories: 195 | Carbohydrates: 25 g | Protein: 1 g | Fat: 10 g | Cholesterol: 156 mg

69. LEMON CHEESECAKE SMOOTHIE

Prep Time: 5 minutes
Cook Time: 5 minutes
Total Time: 10 minutes
Servings: 2

Ingredients:
- 1 medium juicy lemon
- 1 cup (240 mls) light canned coconut milk
- ¼ heaping cup (50 grams) cooked chickpeas
- 1 to 2 Medjool dates
- ¼ cup (25 grams) chopped pecan measured in pieces, not whole
- 1 cup (150 grams) frozen mango pieces
- ¼ teaspoon ground turmeric
- ¼ teaspoon salt
- ½ teaspoon apple cider vinegar
- 1 tablespoon maple syrup optional

Directions:
1. To begin, zest the lemon. Blend the lemon zest, then remove the remaining peel and pith (the white stuff) from the lemon. I do this by cutting both sharp ends of the lemon and then standing it up on the board. Then, with a sharp knife, I sliced all the way around it, just deep enough to remove the pith while leaving the flesh intact.
2. After that, place the entire lemon in the blender and remove the pith and peel.
3. Except for the maple syrup, combine all of the remaining ingredients in a mixing bowl.
4. Blend until the mixture is totally smooth. It yields a thick smoothie. If you like it a little thinner, add a little extra coconut milk or a drop of water to thin it out.
5. If you want a little extra sweetness, add a little more maple syrup. It goes well with maple syrup. Blend for a second on low to disperse, then pour into a glass and serve.

Nutrition Facts: Calories: 549 | Carbohydrates: 68 g | Protein: 6 g | Fat: 39 g | Cholesterol: 140 mg

70. DOUBLE CHOCOLATE SCONES

Prep Time: 10 minutes
Cook Time: 25 minutes
Total Time: 35 minutes
Servings: 8

Ingredients:
- 125g | 1 cup all-purpose flour
- 97g | 3/4 cup wholewheat flour
- 25g | 1/4 cup cocoa powder
- 62g | 1/4 heaping cup natural cane sugar (you can sub this for any granulated sugar or coconut sugar)
- 1/2 teaspoon salt
- 1 tablespoon ground flax
- 1 tablespoon baking powder
- 1/4 packed cup coconut oil (it needs to be hard)
- 1 teaspoon vanilla extract
- 207mls | 3/4 cup + 2 tablespoons cup of non-dairy milk
- 130g | 3/4 cup dairy-free chocolate chips or chunks (I like to use semi-sweet, but you can use any kind you have to hand).
- A little sugar for sprinkling

For the drizzle (optional)
- 43g | 1/4 cup dairy-free chocolate
- 2 tablespoons non-dairy milk

Directions:
1. Pre-heat the oven to 400°F.
2. Use parchment paper or a silicone baking mat to line a baking sheet.
3. In a large mixing basin, combine the flour and baking powder.
4. Mix in the coconut oil with your fingertips or a pastry cutter until the mixture resembles bread crumbs.
5. Stir in all of the remaining dry ingredients, including the chocolate.
6. Add the vanilla extract to the milk and mix to blend, then add the liquid to the dry ingredients and swirl to combine.
7. It's now simpler to get your hands into the dough and shape it into a ball. Don't be too rough with it since the less you handle it, the better your scones will be.
8. Place on the prepared tray and press or roll into a 1 inch thick round.
9. Divide the mixture into 8 equal wedges and divide them so that they all have some space between them.

10. Sprinkle with sugar and bake for 20 - 25 minutes, or until cooked through (if you're not sure, insert a toothpick or skewer and it should come out largely clean).
11. Allow cooling on a cooling rack.
12. Optional chocolate drizzling
13. Place the chocolate and milk in a small dish and gently melt in a microwave or over a saucepan of boiling water.
14. Drizzle the melted chocolate mixture over the cooled scones using a spoon.

Nutrition Facts: Calories: 285 | Carbohydrates: 41 g | Protein: 6 g | Fat: 12 g | Cholesterol: 90 mg

CHAPTER 6: LUNCH (CLEAR FLUIDS)

71. TROPICAL SMOOTHIE (PINEAPPLE, PAPAYA, COCONUT, LIME SMOOTHIE)

Prep Time: 9 minutes
Cook Time: 10 minutes
Total Time: 19 minutes
Servings: 2

Ingredients:
- 1/2 cup coconut water
- 2 tablespoons fresh lime juice
- 1 cup fresh pineapple (chopped)
- 1 cup chopped papaya
- 1 frozen banana (roughly chopped)
- 8 ice cubes

Directions:
1. In the jar of a KitchenAid® Pro Line® Blender, add coconut water, lime juice, pineapple, papaya, banana, and ice in the order listed. Secure the top and turn the blender to the Smoothie setting. Blend until the machine shuts down.
2. Alternatively, put all of the ingredients in a blender, seal the cover, and set the dial to Speed 1. Gradually increase the speed to high (Speed 10 or 11). Blend for 1 minute or until totally smooth. If required, use a Flex Edge tamper to scrape down the jar's sides.
3. Smoothies taste best when served immediately.

Nutrition Facts: Calories: 201 | Carbohydrates: 51 g | Protein: 8 g | Fat: 6 g | Cholesterol: 149 mg

72. CHICKEN BROTH

Prep Time: 60 minutes
Cook Time: 360 minutes
Total Time: 420 minutes
Servings: 12

Ingredients:
- 1 3-4 pounds Whole Chicken
- 12 Cups Water
- 1 tablespoon Olive Oil Extra Virgin
- 1 Medium Onion Peeled and Chopped
- 1 Bunch Celery, including leafy bits Chopped
- 1 Pound Carrots Peeled and Chopped
- 1 Medium Turnip Peeled and Chopped
- 1 Pound Parsnip Peeled and Chopped
- 1 Bunch Dill
- 1 Bunch Parsley
- 1 tablespoon Salt
- 1 tablespoon Pepper

Directions:
1. In a large stockpot over medium heat, heat the olive oil. Cook for 2 minutes, frequently stirring, after adding the onions.
2. Cook for 5-10 minutes, often stirring, until the carrots and celery begin to soften.
3. Cook for another 5-10 minutes, or until the parsnips and turnips are tender and slightly caramelized.
4. Remove the gizzards of the chicken and open the package. Cool water should be used to wash the bird both inside and out.
5. Place the chicken in the pan on top of the veggies. Fill halfway with water. If you like, you may add extra water to make more broth.
6. To the water, add the salt, fresh dill, and fresh parsley. Bring the water to a boil.
7. Reduce the heat to low and simmer for 4-5 hours, or until the chicken is fully cooked and the veggies are tender. Stirring every now and again
8. Remove the chicken from the water with care.
9. Place another stock pot in the sink and cover with a colander. Pour the stock and veggies through the colander, being careful not to get any pieces of vegetables or herbs into the stock.

10. If you have family members who aren't having bariatric surgery, you could shred the chicken, combine it with the veggies and some fresh peas and corn, and use the leftovers to make a chicken pot pie. Otherwise, you may throw them away.

Nutrition Facts: Calories: 163 | Carbohydrates: 27 g | Protein: 7 g | Fat: 4 g | Cholesterol: 276 mg

73. CHICKEN DETOX SOUP

Prep Time: 20 minutes
Cook Time: 35 minutes
Total Time: 55 minutes
Servings: 12

Ingredients:
- 1 1/2 pounds boneless skinless chicken breast
- 2 quarts chicken broth
- 1 large onion, peeled and chopped
- 3 cups broccoli florets
- 2 1/2 cups sliced carrots
- 2 cups chopped celery
- 1 1/2 cups frozen peas
- 1/4 cup chopped parsley
- 3 tablespoons fresh ginger, shredded or grated
- 4 garlic cloves minced
- 2 tablespoons olive oil
- 1 tablespoon apple cider vinegar
- 1/4 teaspoon ground turmeric
- salt

Directions:
1. Preheat a large sauce pot to medium heat. Combine the olive oil, chopped onions, celery, ginger, and garlic in a mixing bowl. Soften for 5-6 minutes in a hot pan. Then combine the raw chicken breasts, broth, carrots, apple cider vinegar, turmeric, and 1 teaspoon sea salt in a mixing bowl.
2. Bring to a boil, then reduce to low heat and cook for 20 minutes, or until the chicken breasts are cooked through. Then, using tongs, take the chicken and place it on a chopping board to cool.
3. To the saucepan, add broccoli, peas, and parsley. Simmer for another 5 minutes to soften the broccoli. Meanwhile, using two forks, shred the chicken breasts and mix them back into the soup. When the broccoli is cooked, taste it and season with salt to suit. Serve hot.

Nutrition Facts: Calories: 91 | Carbohydrates: 6 g | Protein: 9 g | Fat: 2 g | Cholesterol: 24 mg

74. BANANA OAT SHAKE

Prep Time: 20 minutes
Cook Time: 0 minutes
Total Time: 20 minutes
Servings: 2

Ingredients:
- 1/2 cup cooked oatmeal, chilled
- 2/3 cup skim milk
- 2 tablespoons brown sugar
- 1 tablespoon wheat germ
- 1 1/2 teaspoons vanilla extract
- 1/2 frozen banana, cut into chunks

Directions:
1. Blend the oatmeal for a few minutes in a blender.
2. Mix in the milk, brown sugar, wheat germ, vanilla extract, and 1/2 banana. Blend until the mixture is thick and smooth.
3. If desired, serve with ice.

Nutrition Facts: Calories: 173 | Carbohydrates: 33 g | Protein: 6 g | Fat: 1 g | Cholesterol: 150 mg

75. BANANA-APPLE SMOOTHIE

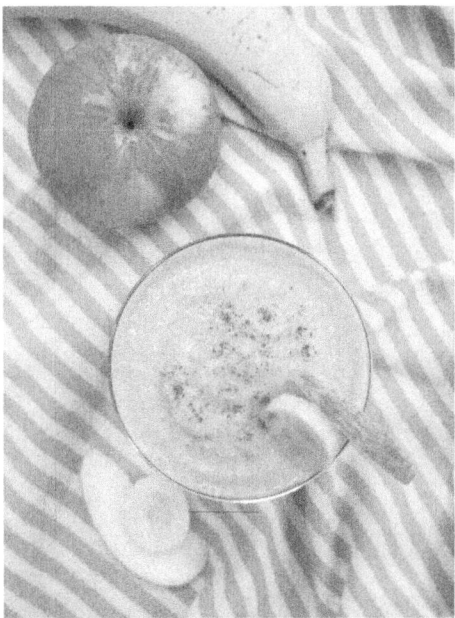

Prep Time: 15 minutes
Cook Time: 0 minutes
Total Time: 15 minutes
Servings: 1

Ingredients:
- 1/2 banana, peeled & cut into chunks
- 1/2 cup plain yogurt
- 1/2 cup unsweetened applesauce
- 1/4 cup skim milk
- 1 tablespoon honey
- 2 tablespoons oat bran

Directions:
1. In a blender, combine the banana, yogurt, applesauce, milk, and honey.
2. Blend until completely smooth.
3. Blend in the oat bran until it is thickened.

Nutrition Facts: Calories: 292 | Carbohydrates: 61 g | Protein: 9 g | Fat: 17 g | Cholesterol: 103 mg

76. BERRYLICIOUS SMOOTHIE

Prep Time: 20 minutes
Cook Time: 0 minutes
Total Time: 20 minutes
Servings: 2

Ingredients:
- 1/4 cup cranberry juice cocktail
- 2/3 cup silken tofu, firm
- 1/2 cup raspberries, frozen, unsweetened
- 1/2 cup blueberries, frozen, unsweetened
- 1 teaspoon vanilla extract
- 1/2 teaspoon powdered lemonade, such as Country Time

Directions:
1. Fill a blender halfway with juice.
2. Combine the remaining ingredients.
3. Blend until completely smooth.
4. Serve right away and enjoy!

Nutrition Facts: Calories: 115 | Carbohydrates: 18 g | Protein: 6 g | Fat: 3 g | Cholesterol: 223 mg

77. BUTTERMILK HERB RANCH DRESSING

Prep Time: 10 minutes
Cook Time: 0 minutes
Total Time: 10 minutes
Servings: 2

Ingredients:
- 1/2 cup mayonnaise
- 1/2 cup milk
- 2 tablespoons vinegar
- 1 tablespoon fresh chives, chopped
- 1 tablespoon dill
- 1 tablespoon oregano leaves, chopped
- 1/4 teaspoon garlic powder

Directions:
1. In a medium mixing dish, combine mayonnaise, milk, and vinegar.
2. Then, with 1/4 teaspoon garlic powder, add fresh chives, dill, and oregano leaves.
3. Combine everything.
4. Allow at least one hour for flavors to emerge.

5. Before serving, thoroughly mix the dressing.

Nutrition Facts: Calories: 83 | Carbohydrates: 1 g | Protein: 1 g | Fat: 6 g | Cholesterol: 64 mg
Nutrition Facts

78. **CITRUS RELISH**

Prep Time: 10 minutes
Cook Time: 2 minutes
Total Time: 12 minutes
Servings: 8

Ingredients:
- 2 pounds small lemons, limes, kumquats or oranges
- 1-quart white vinegar
- 1/4 cup mustard
- glass jars
- 2-4 tablespoons sugar

Directions:
Pickled Fruit
1. At the stem end of each fruit, make a cross. Quarter the oranges if using.
2. Fill glass jars halfway with vinegar.
3. To each jar, add 2 tablespoons of mustard. Put on the lids.
4. Allow it to sit at room temperature for about a month before preparing the relish listed below and serving.

Citrus Relish
1. In a small frying pan, combine the fruit and sugar; add additional sugar to taste.
2. 5-10 minutes, shake the pan often over medium heat until the mixture boils and the fruit turns glossy and transparent.
3. Serve hot or cold.
4. The vinegar left over from the pickled fruit can be used to make salad dressing or to marinade chicken or seafood.

Nutrition Facts: Calories: 26 | Carbohydrates: 7 g | Protein: 0 g | Fat: 0 g | Cholesterol: 37 mg

79. **CHICKPEA PANCAKES RECIPE**

Prep Time: 10 minutes
Cook Time: 15 minutes
Total Time: 25 minutes
Servings: 23

Ingredients:
- 1 cup (120g) Chickpea Flour
- 1 1/2 cups 375ml Water
- 2 tablespoon Olive Oil *See Note 1
- 1 Carrot, finely grated
- 1/4 Red Capsicum, finely chopped
- 1 Spring Onion, finely chopped
- 1/4 tablespoon Turmeric
- 1/4 tablespoon Cumin
- 2 tablespoon Chopped Coriander (cilantro)
- 1/4 tablespoon Salt

Directions:
7. In a mixing basin, combine the chickpea flour and water, constantly stirring to create a smooth, lump-free batter. Set aside.
8. Heat 1/2 tablespoon of the oil in a frying pan over medium-high heat. Combine the carrot, onion, turmeric, and cumin in a mixing bowl. Reduce the heat to medium-low and continue to simmer until the vegetables are softened (around 4-5 mins)
9. Combine the carrot mixture, chopped coriander, and salt in the chickpea batter (if using). Stir until everything is well mixed.
10. Over medium-high heat, heat a nonstick frying pan. When the pan is heated, pour in the olive oil (or alternatively, use spray oil). Place a tablespoon of batter in the pan and spread it out with the back of your spoon (to make them thinner). To fill the pan, repeat the process. (*Please see Note 3)
11. Cook each side for about 2 minutes (this will vary depending on the pan, heat, and how thin your pancake is). Look for bubbles to develop (as seen above), and your pancakes should be able to be easily flipped.

12. Remove the pancakes from the pan and continue with the rest of the batter.

Nutrition Facts: Calories: 32 | Carbohydrates: 3 g | Protein: 1 g | Fat: 1 g | Cholesterol: 27 mg

80. RED WINE SANGRIA RECIPE

Prep Time: 15 minutes
Cook Time: 15 minutes
Total Time: 30 minutes
Servings: 8

Ingredients:
- 750 ml Rioja wine
- 3/4 cup Solerno blood orange liqueur
- 3/4 cup Leblon Cachaca Brazilian rum
- 1 1/2 cup orange juice
- 3/4 cup cherry juice
- 3/4 cup simple syrup sugar syrup
- 1/2 cup fresh lime juice
- 1 1/2 cups watermelon balls
- 1 cup raspberries
- 1 cup blackberries
- 2 mandarin oranges sliced
- 1 lime sliced
- 1 bunch basil leaves

Directions:
1. Stir together all of the liquid ingredients in a large pitcher. Then, to the pitcher, add the fresh fruit.
2. Refrigerate for at least 2 hours, covered. Pour into glasses and garnish with fresh basil leaves when ready to serve.

Nutrition Facts: Calories: 360 | Carbohydrates: 51 g | Protein: 1 g | Fat: 1 g | Cholesterol: 423 mg

81. SALTY DOG COCKTAIL RECIPE

Prep Time: 3 minutes
Cook Time: 0 minutes
Total Time: 3 minutes
Servings: 2

Ingredients:
- Four oz ruby red grapefruit juice
- Two oz vodka
- One ounce club soda or sparkling grapefruit-flavored water
- 1-2 teaspoons simple syrup
- Ice
- For Garnish: Kosher salt or Fleur de Sel agave syrup, grapefruit wedges

Directions:
1. Set out two tiny shallow plates for the Salt Rim. In one plate, spread salt, and in the other, spread a thin layer of agave syrup (or just syrup). Dip the edge of a highball glass in the syrup before dipping it in the salt.
2. Fill the glass three-quarters full of ice for each cocktail. Combine the grapefruit juice, vodka, club soda, and 1 teaspoon simple syrup in a mixing bowl.
3. Use a cocktail swizzle stick to stir. If desired, add a bit extra simple syrup to taste. Serve with a fresh grapefruit slice on the rim.

Notes: Add a sprinkle of cayenne to the salt before dipping for a fiery Salty Dog.

Nutrition Facts: Calories: 202 | Carbohydrates: 18 g | Protein: 1 g | Fat: 11 g | Cholesterol: 26 mg

82. SIMPLE SYRUP

Prep Time: 2 minutes
Cook Time: 3 minutes
Total Time: 5 minutes
Servings: 8

Ingredients:
- 1 cup water
- 1 cup granulated sugar or turbinado, demerara

Directions:
1. Heat a small saucepot on high. Fill the saucepan halfway with water and sugar.

2. Bring to a boil, stirring constantly. Once boiling, remove from heat and stir. (If using herbs for infusion, add them to the simple boiling syrup.)
3. Allow cooling to room temperature before storing in an airtight container.

Nutrition Facts: Calories: 97 | Carbohydrates: 25 g | Protein: 2 g | Fat: 12 g | Cholesterol: 44 mg

83. ROSE SANGRIA RECIPE

Prep Time: 15 minutes
Cook Time: 0 minutes
Total Time: 15 minutes
Servings: 8

Ingredients:
- 750 ml French Rosé Wine (1 bottle)
- 1 cup pink grapefruit juice
- 3/4 cup bourbon
- 1/2 cup honey
- 1/4 cup Chambord (raspberry liqueur)
- 2 cups watermelon balls
- 1 1/2 cups fresh sliced strawberries
- 6 oz fresh raspberries

Directions:
1. Scoop 2 cups of watermelon balls from a big piece of fresh watermelon using a melon baller. Strawberries, sliced
2. In a large pitcher, combine the rosé wine, grapefruit juice, whiskey, honey, and Chambord. Stir the honey into the mixture until it melts. (If your honey is particularly thick, reheat it first to thin it up before adding to the recipe.) After that, toss in the watermelon balls and strawberries. Refrigerate for at least 2 hours, covered.
3. Stir and taste for sweetness after at least two hours. If you want your sangria sweeter, add a bit, extra honey. If the sangria is too powerful, serve it over ice. When ready to serve, mix in the fresh raspberries and divide among glasses.

Nutrition Facts: Calories: 209 | Carbohydrates: 26 g | Protein: 0 g | Fat: 0 g | Cholesterol: 180 mg

84. CHAMPAGNE HOLIDAY PUNCH RECIPE

Prep Time: 2 minutes
Cook Time: 5 minutes
Total Time: 7 minutes
Servings: 16

Ingredients:
- 750 ml of champagne (1 bottle)
- 24 oz ginger beer (2 bottles)
- Three cups of cranberry juice cocktail (or juice blend)
- Two cups of ruby red grapefruit juice
- One cup of spiced rum, optional
- Possible Garnishes: fresh cranberries, grapefruit slices, cinnamon sticks

Directions:
1. All ingredients should be chilled. When ready to serve, combine all of the ingredients in a punch bowl.
2. Serve with cranberries, grapefruit slices, and cinnamon sticks as garnish.

Nutrition Facts: Calories: 107 | Carbohydrates: 13 g | Protein: 0 g | Fat: 0 g | Cholesterol: 0 mg

85. WHITE SANGRIA

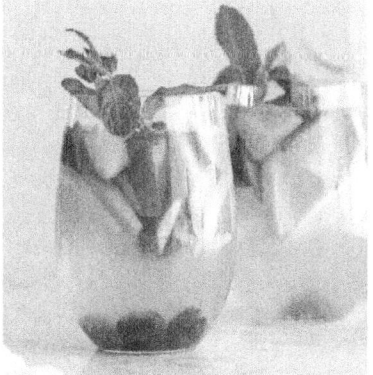

Prep Time: 10 minutes
Cook Time: 10 minutes
Total Time: 20 minutes
Servings: 10

Ingredients:
- 750 ml Moscato wine Riesling is my second choice

- 1 1/2 cups orange-pineapple juice
- 1 cup Domaine de Canton ginger liqueur
- 1/2 cup Midori melon liqueur
- 1 cup cantaloupe balls
- 1 cup sliced strawberries
- 2 mandarin oranges sliced
- 1 lime sliced
- 1-liter club soda chilled

Directions:
1. In a large pitcher, combine the wine, juice, and liqueurs. Refrigerate for at least 1 hour after adding the fruit.
2. Pour into glasses 2/3 full (scoop in some fruit) and top with club soda when ready to serve. Serve chilled.

Nutrition Facts: Calories: 218 | Carbohydrates: 27 g | Protein: 1 g | Fat: 1 g | Cholesterol: 18 mg

86. RASPBERRY MOJITOS WITH BASIL

Prep Time: 10 minutes
Cook Time: 10 minutes
Total Time: 20 minutes
Servings: 8

Ingredients:
- One cup simple syrup 3/4 cup sugar + 3/4 cup water, heated to dissolve
- 1/2 cup torn basil leaves
- One cup FRESH key lime juice use regular limes for slightly less acidity
- One cup white rum
- 1/4 cup Chambord raspberry liquor
- 1-liter club soda
- Ice
- Fresh raspberries and lime slices to garnish

Directions:
1. In a large pitcher, combine the simple cooled syrup and the torn basil leaves. Muddle the basil leaves with a big spoon/ladle to unleash their flavor—beat them up quite hard.
2. Combine the lime juice, rum, and Chambord in a mixing glass. Stir. Stir in the club soda and top with ice if the pitcher permits.
3. Garnish each glass with fresh berries and lime slices to serve. Serve cold with or without ice.

Nutrition Facts: Calories: 283 | Carbohydrates: 36 g | Protein: 1 g | Fat: 1 g | Cholesterol: 53 mg

87. MARGARITA RECIPE

Prep Time: 10 minutes
Cook Time: 10 minutes
Total Time: 20 minutes
Servings: 10

Ingredients:
- 18 oz Tequila Blanco
- 18 oz fresh-squeezed lime juice (could be fresh bottled lime juice from the refrigerated section, but not the concentrated kind. FRESH)
- Nine oz La Belle or Grand Marnier
- Eight oz simple syrup + a little extra for glass rims
- Three oz orange juice
- Three oz Triple Sec
- Coarse or flake sea salt for glass rims
- Sliced lime and orange for garnish

Directions:
1. If you don't have any on hand, start by preparing some simple syrup. 7 oz sugar and 7 oz water Microwave until the sugar is completely dissolved. You should have around 9-10 oz left over for rimming the glasses.
2. Combine all of the margarita ingredients in a big pitcher. Chill after thoroughly stirring.
3. Pour the simple leftover syrup into a shallow dish when ready to serve. In a second shallow dish, add sea salt (or flake salt). Then, dip the rims of the glasses in simple syrup, followed by salt.

4. If preferred, add ice to the glasses, and fill a shaker halfway with ice. Shake the margarita mix for 10-15 seconds in a shaker. Pour into serving glasses. Serve the cups garnished with cut limes or oranges. Ole'!

Nutrition Facts: Calories: 300 | Carbohydrates: 32 g | Protein: 0 g | Fat: 0 g | Cholesterol: 29 mg

88. PINK GRAPEFRUIT MARGARITA

Prep Time: 5 minutes
Cook Time: 5 minutes
Total Time: 10 minutes
Servings: 2

Ingredients:

- Five oz of freshly squeezed ruby red grapefruit juice
- Four oz white tequila
- 1 1/2 oz of Triple Sec orange liquor
- 1/2 ounce of agave syrup + extra for glass rims
- Fresh grapefruit slices for garnish
- Salt for rim

Directions:

1. Put a little quantity of agave syrup on one plate and salt on another. Dip the rims of the glasses first in the syrup, then in the salt. Fill the cups halfway with ice and set them aside.
2. Half-fill a cocktail shaker with ice and mix vigorously. Fill the shaker halfway with fresh grapefruit juice, tequila, Triple Sec, and agave.
3. Cover and vigorously shake for 30 seconds. After that, pour into the glasses. Enjoy with fresh grapefruit slices as a garnish!

Nutrition Facts: Calories: 251 | Carbohydrates: 20 g | Protein: 1 g | Fat: 1 g | Cholesterol: 115 mg

89. GRAPEFRUIT BASIL SORBET

Prep Time: 35 minutes
Cook Time: 20 minutes
Total Time: 55 minutes
Servings: 6

Ingredients:

- Four large ruby red grapefruits, juiced
- Two cups of water
- 1 3/4 cups of organic cane sugar or palm sugar
- Two lemons, zested and juiced
- One cup of basil leaves, packed
- pinch salt

Directions:

1. In a small saucepan, bring the water and sugar to a boil. When the water is boiling, add the lemon zest, basil leaves, and salt. Remove from the heat and cover with a lid. For at least 20 minutes, steep the basil leaves in the simple syrup.
2. Meanwhile, fill a 4-cup measuring pitcher halfway with lemon juice. Juice the grapefruits into the pitcher until 3 glasses of combined juices are measured.
3. Remove the basil leaves and strain the simple syrup. Then combine the syrup and the juice. Refrigerate for at least 2-3 hours (or to speed up, put in the freezer for 1 hour.)
4. Fill an electric ice cream maker halfway with the sorbet mixture. Turn on and mix for at least 20 minutes, or until the mixture achieves a "soft-serve" consistency.
5. Sorbet may be eaten right away or frozen in an airtight container. Allow the sorbet to soften for 10-15 minutes after it has been frozen before serving.

Note: To achieve the brightest, freshest flavor, use freshly squeezed grapefruits rather than pre-squeezed grapefruit juice.

Nutrition Facts: Calories: 272 | Carbohydrates: 70 g | Protein: 1 g | Fat: 1 g | Cholesterol: 38 mg

90. BRULEED GRAPEFRUIT (PAMPLEMOUSSE BRÛLÉ)

Prep Time: 5 minutes
Cook Time: 8 minutes
Total Time: 13 minutes
Servings: 8

Ingredients:
- 4 large ripe ruby red grapefruits
- 8 teaspoons granulated sugar
- Brulee Torch

Directions:
1. Place your index finger on the top of a grapefruit stem and cup your palm around it from top to bottom. Then, cut it in half in the middle. (If you don't notice a floral pattern, you've chopped the grapefruit the incorrect way.) Cut each grapefruit in this manner.
2. I am using a tiny serrated knife cut along the inside rim of each grapefruit half to separate the fruit from the skin. Then, cut along the membrane between each small triangle section so that each mouthful comes out easily with a spoon. Keep everything intact.
3. Sprinkle 1 teaspoon of granulated sugar over the top of each grapefruit half, one at a time. Then, hold the flame over the grapefruit and brulee the top until the sugar turns golden and has candied the top of each half. This should take 30-60 seconds per half. Serve immediately and repeat.

Nutrition Facts: Calories: 67 | Carbohydrates: 12 g | Protein: 2 g | Fat: 2 g | Cholesterol: 86 mg

91. FROZEN BEERITAS RECIPE

Prep Time: 5 minutes
Cook Time: 5 minutes
Total Time: 10 minutes
Servings: 2

Ingredients:
- 3 oz tequila Blanco
- oz Triple Sec (orange liqueur)
- 3 oz fresh lime juice
- 3 oz simple syrup
- 2 oz orange juice
- 14 oz Mexican beer, such as two 7-ounce Coronitas or one 12-ounce can any Mexican beer
- 3-4 cups ice

Directions:
Self-Serve Method
1. In a blender, combine tequila, Triple Sec, lime juice, simple syrup, and orange juice. Pour with 3 glasses of ice. Puree the mixture until it is smooth and foamy. Serve the margaritas in two big tumblers, with a Coronita on the side. As they sip their Margarita, each individual can add beer to it.

Mixed Batch Method
2. In a blender, combine the tequila, Triple Sec, lime juice, simple syrup, orange juice, and a 12-ounce lager. Pour with 4 glasses of ice. Puree the mixture until it is smooth and foamy. Pour into serving glasses and serve.

Nutrition Facts: Calories: 386 | Carbohydrates: 51 g | Protein: 1 g | Fat: 0 g | Cholesterol: 55 mg

92. SPICY PINEAPPLE HABANERO MARGARITAS

Prep Time: 5 minutes
Cook Time: 5 minutes
Total Time: 10 minutes
Servings: 6

Ingredients:
- 1 cup tequila silver
- 1 cup triple sec
- 1 cup fresh-squeezed lime juice
- 2 1/2 cups pineapple juice
- 4 habanero chiles

- Optional garnishes: salt, limes, habaneros, pineapple slices

Directions:
1. Melt the butter in a small pan over medium heat. Remove the from the habaneros by cutting them in half. Place the chiles in the skillet and cook until they are blistered on both sides. Remove from the heat.
2. In a pitcher, combine the tequila, triple sec, lime juice, and pineapple juice. Stir everything together thoroughly.
3. Toss in the blistered habaneros. Allow them to soak in the margarita mix for 15 minutes to overnight. The longer they soak in the mixture, the hotter it will get. After 15 minutes, taste the mixture to see how long you want to soak them. When the heat level is to your taste, remove the habaneros.
4. Pour the margaritas into glasses with ice when ready to serve. Garnish with lime wedges, pineapple slices, or more habaneros if desired.

Nutrition Facts: Calories: 287 | Carbohydrates: 31 g | Protein: 1 g | Fat: 0 g | Cholesterol: 65 mg

93. CRANBERRY POMEGRANATE MARGARITA WITH SPICED RIM

Prep Time: 5 minutes
Cook Time: 5 minutes
Total Time: 10 minutes
Servings: 4

Ingredients:
- 2 cups cranberry pomegranate juice blend
- 2 cups Tequila Blanco
- 1 cup fresh squeezed lime juice
- 1/2 cup triple sec
- 2 tablespoons coarse sea salt
- 1 teaspoon Old El Paso Taco Seasoning
- 2 tablespoons agave syrup

Directions:
1. 1 tablespoon water and 1 tablespoon agave syrup on a dish To combine, gently mix everything together.
2. On a separate dish, combine the salt and Old El Paso Taco Seasoning.
3. Using the agave syrup, coat the rims of 4-6 glasses. Then, dip the rims in the seasoned salt. Fill the cups halfway with ice.
4. In a large ice-filled shaker or pitcher, combine the cranberry pomegranate juice, tequila, lime juice, and triple sec. Shake or mix before pouring into glasses and serving!

Nutrition Facts: Calories: 483 | Carbohydrates: 38 g | Protein: 0 g | Fat: 0 g | Cholesterol: 346 mg

94. PEACH MILKSHAKE (COPYCAT CHIK-FIL-A PEACH SHAKE RECIPE!)

Prep Time: 5 minutes
Cook Time: 5 minutes
Total Time: 10 minutes
Servings: 4

Ingredients:
- 6 ripe peaches pitted, skins on
- 7 scoops of vanilla ice cream
- 3 tablespoons granulated sugar
- ½ teaspoon vanilla extract
- 1 pinch salt
- Optional: Whipped cream and maraschino cherries

Directions:
1. Remove the pits from the peaches and cut them in half.
2. Combine the peaches, ice cream, sugar, vanilla, and salt in a large blender.
3. Puree till smooth, covered.

Nutrition Facts: Calories: 397 | Carbohydrates: 62 g | Protein: 7 g | Fat: 9 g | Cholesterol: 14 mg

95. JUGO VERDE (GREEN JUICE)

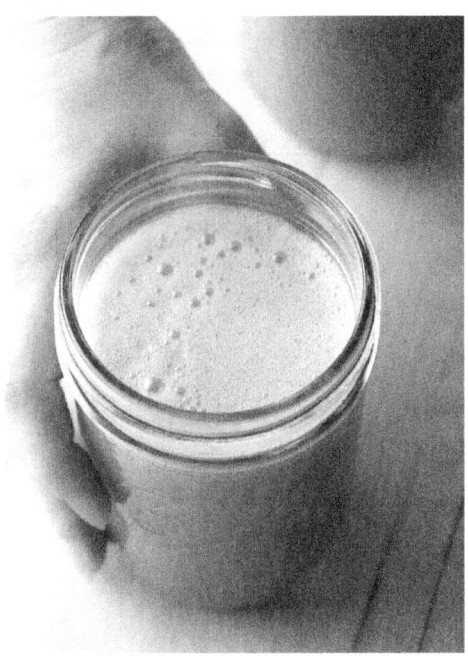

Prep Time: 10 minutes
Cook Time: 0 minutes
Total Time: 10 minutes
Servings: 5

Ingredients:
- 2 cups orange juice
- 1 1/2 cups fresh pineapple chunks
- 1/2 Nopal cactus paddle chopped (or substitute 1 celery stalk)
- 1 large cucumber with peel, cut into chunks
- 1/4 cup packed parsley or cilantro

Directions:
1. In a blender, combine all of the ingredients. Add a bit of salt, close the lid tightly, and puree until smooth.
2. When the mixture is green and frothy, serve immediately or strain over a screen to remove the pulp.

Nutrition Facts: Calories: 67 | Carbohydrates: 12 g | Protein: 2 g | Fat: 2 g | Cholesterol: 86 mg

96. PERFECT MANHATTAN RECIPE

Prep Time: 2 minutes
Cook Time: 5 minutes
Total Time: 7 minutes
Servings: 1

Ingredients:
- 2 oz bourbon or rye whiskey
- 1-ounce sweet vermouth like Antica
- 2 dashes of angostura bitters
- Garnishes: twist of lemon rind, orange rind, or a maraschino cherry

Directions:
1. Fill a cocktail shaker halfway with ice for each Manhattan Cocktail. Combine the bourbon, sweet vermouth, and bitters in a mixing glass.
2. Using a bar spoon, stir everything together. Don't jiggle. Then strain into a coupe cocktail glass or a low ball glass filled with ice.
3. Serve with a maraschino cherry, lemon peel twist, or orange rind twist as a garnish.

Nutrition Facts: Calories: 190 | Carbohydrates: 2 g | Protein: 1 g | Fat: 16 g | Cholesterol: 293 mg

97. FROZEN COCONUT MOJITO

Prep Time: 5 minutes
Cook Time: 5 minutes
Total Time: 10 minutes
Servings: 2

Ingredients:
- 4 oz cream of coconut
- 4 oz coconut rum
- 2 oz fresh lime juice
- 8 fresh mint leaves
- 4 cups ice

Directions:

1. In a high-powered blender, combine all of the ingredients with 4 cups of ice. Pour into glasses after blending until totally smooth.
2. If desired, garnish with mint and lime slices.

Nutrition Facts: Calories: 386 | Carbohydrates: 43 g | Protein: 1 g | Fat: 9 g | Cholesterol: 182 mg

98. MULLED LEMONADE RECIPE

Prep Time: 20 minutes
Cook Time: 5 minutes
Total Time: 25 minutes
Servings: 8

Ingredients:
- 5 cups water divided
- 1 cup granulated sugar
- 1 cup fresh lemon juice
- 3 cinnamon sticks
- 6 whole star anise
- 4 slices fresh ginger
- 4 pieces orange peel large
- 20 whole cloves
- 6 cracked green cardamom pods
- 1/2 teaspoon pink peppercorns

Directions:
1. 2 cups of water, brought to a boil Mix in the sugar and all of the pieces. Allow the simple syrup to steep for at least 20 minutes, covered. (The more time you have, the better.)
2. Fill a big pitcher halfway with syrup. Then add the remaining three cups of water and lemon juice. Fill the pitcher halfway with ice and swirl well.

Notes: If you don't want "floaties" in your drinks, drain the spices out of the simple syrup.

Nutrition Facts: Calories: 117 | Carbohydrates: 30 g | Protein: 1 g | Fat: 1 g | Cholesterol: 70 mg

99. CUCUMBER ROSE APEROL SPRITZ

Prep Time: 5 minutes
Cook Time: 5 minutes
Total Time: 10 minutes
Servings: 1

Ingredients:
- oz rose-infused Aperol*
- 2 oz sparkling wine such as Prosecco
- 2 slices cucumber about an inch thick
- Splash club soda

Directions:
1. To make rose-infused Aperol, mix one 750ml bottle Aperol with one ounce dried rose petals (these can be found in the bulk section of most specialty food stores). Shake everything together and set it aside for a few hours or overnight. After straining off the rose petals, the Aperol is ready to use.
2. In a cocktail shaker, combine the Rose Aperol and cucumber with ice. Fill a tall Collins glass halfway with ice and strain it into it. Pour in the sparkling wine and ice. Garnish with fresh cucumber and a dash of club soda.

Nutrition Facts: Calories: 143 | Carbohydrates: 12 g | Protein: 1 g | Fat: 1 g | Cholesterol: 50 mg

100. PINK GRAPEFRUIT MARGARITA

Prep Time: 5 minutes
Cook Time: 0 minutes
Total Time: 5 minutes
Servings: 2

Ingredients:
- Five oz of freshly squeezed ruby red grapefruit juice
- Four oz of white tequila
- 1 1/2 oz of Triple Sec orange liquor
- 1/2 ounce of agave syrup + extra for glass rims
- Fresh grapefruit slices for garnish
- Salt for rim

Directions:
1. Put a little quantity of agave syrup on one plate and salt on another. Dip the rims of the glasses first in the syrup, then in the salt. Fill the cups halfway with ice and set them aside.
2. Fill an ice-filled cocktail shaker halfway with ice. Fill the shaker halfway with fresh grapefruit juice, tequila, Triple Sec, and agave.
3. Cover and vigorously shake for 30 seconds. After that, pour into the glasses. Enjoy with fresh grapefruit slices as a garnish!

Nutrition Facts: Calories: 251 | Carbohydrates: 20 g | Protein: 1 g | Fat: 1 g | Cholesterol: 192 mg

101. STRAWBERRY MARGARITA RECIPE

Prep Time: 10 minutes
Cook Time: 0 minutes
Total Time: 10 minutes
Servings: 2

Ingredients:
- 1 pound fresh strawberries, trimmed
- 1 cup tequila
- 3/4 cup fresh lime juice
- 2/3 cup strawberry jam
- 1/4 cup triple sec
- 10 mint leaves
- 3-4 cups ice
- Optional Garnish: margarita salt, lime slices, extra strawberries

Directions:
1. Prepare a big blender. Add the fresh-cut strawberries, tequila, lime juice, strawberry jam, triple sec, mint leaves, and ice to the container.
2. Blend until smooth.
3. Toppings: Paint additional strawberry jam around the rims of four glasses using a pastry brush. Dip the rims of the glasses in margarita salt.
4. Fill the glass halfway with cold margaritas. Serve with a fresh lime slice and a strawberry on top.

Nutrition Facts: Calories: 391 | Carbohydrates: 57 g | Protein: 1 g | Fat: 1 g | Cholesterol: 142 mg

102. LARGE-BATCH GOOMBAY SMASH CARIBBEAN COCKTAILS

Prep Time: 5 minutes
Cook Time: 3 minutes
Total Time: 8 minutes
Servings: 40

Ingredients:
- 14 cups 100% pineapple juice
- 2 bottles of dark Caribbean rum (750 ml each - I used Pusser's)
- 1 bottle coconut rum (750 ml - Cruzan)
- 2 cups fresh-squeezed lime juice
- 1 1/2 cups simple syrup
- 1 cup orange liqueur (Cointreau)
- 1/2 teaspoon bitters, optional
- Fresh pineapple slices for garnish

Directions:
1. If you're creating your own simple syrup, mix 1 cup granulated sugar and 1 cup water. Cook until the sugar melts on the burner. Allow cooling fully.
2. Fill a big beverage dispenser halfway with all of the ingredients. Stir everything together thoroughly. Chill until ready to serve, then top with cut pineapples.
3. Serve with ice.

Nutrition Facts: Calories: 222 | Carbohydrates: 22 g | Protein: 0 g | Fat: 0 g | Cholesterol: 11 mg

103. HEALTHY VEGAN BROWNIES

Prep Time: 15 minutes
Cook Time: 30 minutes
Total Time: 45 minutes
Servings: 9

Ingredients:
- 4 tablespoon ground flax
- ⅔ cup warm water
- 1 cup date sugar or coconut sugar
- 1 cup cacao powder
- ½ cup white whole wheat flour
- ½ tablespoon salt
- 1 tablespoon baking powder
- ½ cup unsweetened applesauce or pumpkin puree
- 1 tablespoon vanilla extract
- ¼ cup unsweetened almond milk optional

Directions:
6. Preheat the oven to 325 degrees Fahrenheit. In a small dish, combine ground flax and warm water. Allow for a 15-minute resting period.
7. In a medium mixing bowl, combine the dry ingredients (date sugar, cacao powder, white whole wheat flour, baking powder, and salt) while the flax egg is setting.
8. In the middle of the dry ingredients, make a well. Combine the wet and dry components (flax egg, applesauce/or pumpkin puree, and vanilla extract). Stir until well mixed. If the batter appears to be too dry, add 14 cups of unsweetened almond milk.
9. Pour the batter into an 8-inch square baking dish lined with parchment paper. Distribute evenly.
10. 30–35 minutes in the oven, or until a toothpick inserted in the middle comes out clean. Allow cooling fully in the pan before removing and cutting into squares.

Nutrition Facts: Calories: 126 | Carbohydrates: 28 g | Protein: 3 g | Fat: 1 g | Cholesterol: 172 mg

104. GREEN CHICKEN SOUP

Prep Time: 15 minutes
Cook Time: 25 minutes
Total Time: 40 minutes
Servings: 12

Ingredients:
- Two quarts of chicken broth or stock
- 1 ½ pound boneless, skinless chicken breast
- Two celery stalks, chopped
- Two cups of green beans, cut into 1-inch pieces
- One and a half cups peas, fresh or frozen
- Two cups asparagus, cut into 1-inch pieces, tops and middles (avoid tough ends)
- One cup of diced green onions
- 4-6 cloves garlic, minced
- Two cups of fresh spinach leaves, chopped and packed
- One bunch watercress, chopped with large stems removed
- 1/2 cup of fresh parsley leaves, chopped
- 1/3 cup of fresh basil leaves, chopped
- One teaspoon salt

Directions:
1. In a large saucepan, boil the chicken broth over medium-high heat. Bring the chicken breasts to a simmer in the sauce. The cooking time is 15 minutes.
2. Combine the celery, green beans, peas, asparagus, onions, garlic, salt in a mixing bowl. Simmer for 5-10 minutes, or until the vegetables are soft, then remove from the heat.
3. Remove the chicken breasts and shred or cut them into bite-sized pieces with two forks. Back to the pot.

4. Combine the spinach, watercress, parsley, and basil in a mixing bowl. Season with salt to taste.

Nutrition Facts: Calories: 105 | Carbohydrates: 7 g | Protein: 15 g | Fat: 2 g | Cholesterol: 134 mg

105. GREEN RISOTTO RECIPE

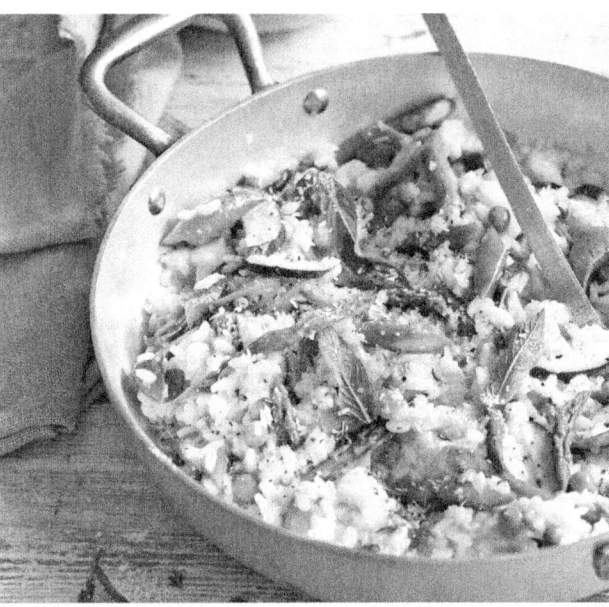

Prep Time: 10 minutes
Cook Time: 40 minutes
Total Time: 50 minutes
Servings: 8

Ingredients:
- Two cups arborio rice
- Three tablespoons butter
- Three tablespoons olive oil
- Six scallions, greens and whites chopped
- Two and a half cups fresh packed spinach leaves
- One cup packed fresh parsley
- 12 fresh basil leaves
- Three garlic cloves
- Six cups chicken broth, room temperature (vegetable broth for vegetarians)
- One cup of white wine
- One cup of shredded parmesan cheese
- Salt

Directions:
1. In a blender, combine spinach, parsley, basil, and garlic. Add 4 cups broth and purée until completely smooth.
2. In a large sauté pan, combine the butter and oil. In a medium saucepan over medium heat, melt the butter. Add the scallions once the butter has melted and cooked for 2 minutes. After adding the rice, cook for another 2 minutes. Then stir in the wine, 1 1/2 teaspoons of salt, and 1/2 teaspoon ground.
3. Simmer, occasionally stirring, until the wine has been absorbed. Start with the 2 cups of liquid that was not put into the blender and add one cup of broth at a time to the rice. Stir the rice after each addition of liquid and let it boil until the broth is absorbed before adding more. Ensure that all of the green herb broth is included in the blender. This procedure will take approximately 25 minutes.
4. Stir in the grated parmesan cheese after you've poured the rest of the green liquid and the rice is cooked but still firm. Turn off the heat before the last round of stock has been completely absorbed, leaving the risotto a bit soupy. As it cools, it will stiffen up. Season to taste with salt and serve warm.

Nutrition Facts: Calories: 283 | Carbohydrates: 36 g | Protein: 1 g | Fat: 1 g | Cholesterol: 53 mg

106. RASPBERRY MOJITOS WITH BASIL

Prep Time: 10 minutes
Cook Time: 10 minutes
Total Time: 20 minutes
Servings: 8

Ingredients:
- One cup of simple syrup 3/4 cup sugar + 3/4 cup water, heated to dissolve

- 1/2 cup torn basil leaves
- One cup of FRESH key lime juice use regular limes for slightly less acidity
- One cup white rum
- 1/4 cup Chambord raspberry liquor
- One liter club soda
- Ice
- Fresh raspberries and lime slices to garnish

Directions:
1. In a large pitcher, combine the simple cooled syrup and the torn basil leaves. Muddle the basil leaves with a big spoon/ladle to unleash their flavor—beat them up quite hard.
2. Combine the lime juice, rum, and Chambord in a mixing glass. Stir. Stir in the club soda and top with ice if the pitcher permits.
3. Garnish each glass with fresh berries and lime slices to serve. Serve cold with or without ice.

Nutrition Facts: Calories: 284 | Carbohydrates: 36 g | Protein: 1 g | Fat: 1 g | Cholesterol: 66 mg

107. DRUNKEN MONKEY COCKTAIL

Prep Time: 3 minutes
Cook Time: 3 minutes
Total Time: 6 minutes
Servings: 1

Ingredients:
- 6 oz orange-pineapple juice blend
- 3 oz coconut rum
- 1 ounce spiced rum
- 4-5 dashes of bitters
- Fresh ground nutmeg
- Maraschino cherries in juices
- Lime slices
- Fresh pineapple wedges

Directions:
1. Pour the juice, coconut rum, spiced rum, and 4-5 shakes of bitters into a cocktail shaker with ice. Shake vigorously for 30 seconds.
2. Pour into two ice-filled tumblers or a large glass. Then add 1-2 tablespoons of cherry juice and let it settle at the bottom of the glass. Garnish with a slice of lime, a wedge of pineapple, and a cherry.
3. Serve with freshly grated nutmeg on top.

Nutrition Facts: Calories: 202 | Carbohydrates: 16 g | Protein: 1 g | Fat: 1 g | Cholesterol: 111 mg

108. NEGRONI RECIPE

Prep Time: 3 minutes
Cook Time: 5 minutes
Total Time: 8 minutes
Servings: 1

Ingredients:
- ¾ ounce Tanqueray No. Ten Gin
- ¾ ounce Dolin Blanc
- ¾ ounce Aperol
- ¾ ounce freshly brewed chamomile tea

Directions:
1. Stir together all of the ingredients with ice and pour into a chilled coupe.
2. Garnish with a grapefruit peel, ensuring that the oil from the peel is extracted and placed on top of the cocktail.

Nutrition Facts: Calories: 123 | Carbohydrates: 7 g | Protein: 1 g | Fat: 2 g | Cholesterol: 86 mg

109. POG PUNCH HAWAIIAN COCKTAIL

Prep Time: 5 minutes
Cook Time: 5 minutes
Total Time: 10 minutes
Servings: 10

Ingredients:
For the POG Juice

- 3 cups pink guava nectar juice
- 3 cups passion fruit juice
- 1 1/2 cups orange juice
- For the POG Punch Hawaiian Cocktail:
- 7 1/2 cups POG juice
- 10 oz Malibu Rum
- 750 ml dry champagne
- Ice
- Fresh tropical fruit for garnish

Directions:
1. Combine the POG juice ingredients in a large punch bowl.
2. Garnish with fresh tropical fruit and rum and champagne. If necessary, add ice.
3. In a glass, combine 3/4 cup POG, 1 ounce Malibu Rum, and 1/3 cup champagne. Stir in the ice.

Nutrition Facts: Calories: 271 | Carbohydrates: 43 g | Protein: 1 g | Fat: 0 g | Cholesterol: 32 mg

110. MULLED WINE (WASSAIL RECIPE)

Prep Time: 3 minutes
Cook Time: 180 minutes
Total Time: 183 minutes
Servings: 12

Ingredients:
- Two bottles of fruity red wine, like a rioja or pinot noir (750ml-bottles)
- Four cups of apple cider
- Two and a half cups orange juice
- 1/2 cup honey
- Two cups frozen pitted cherries
- One large apple of sliced thin into rounds
- One of a large orange, sliced thin into rounds
- 1 piece fresh ginger (2 inches), sliced
- 8-10 cinnamon sticks
- One vanilla bean, cut open from end to end
- One teaspoon cloves

Directions:
1. In a large slow cooker, combine all of the ingredients. Cover and cook for at least 3 hours on high or 5 hours on low.
2. Fill glasses or mugs halfway with hot mulled wine. Garnish with the fruit and cinnamon sticks if desired.

Nutrition Facts: Calories: 137 | Carbohydrates: 35 g | Protein: 0 g | Fat: 0 g | Cholesterol: 1 mg

111. FRENCH LAVENDER LEMONADE RECIPE

Prep Time: 15 minutes
Cook Time: 5 minutes
Total Time: 20 minutes
Servings: 10

Ingredients:
- Ten cups of water, divided
- Three cups of granulated sugar
- 1/2 cup lavender leaves, roughly chopped
- Two cups freshly of squeezed lemon juice, from 9-11 lemons
- Ice
- Fresh lavender sprigs for garnishing

Directions:
1. 5 cups of water, sugar, and lavender leaves in a medium sauce pan. Bring the water to a boil. When the water is boiling, mix it in and cover it. Remove from the heat and let aside to steep until the mixture comes to room temperature.
2. Squeeze the lemons, taking care to remove any stray seeds. Remove the lavender leaves when the simple lavender syrup has cooled. In a large pitcher, combine the syrup, lemon juice, and 5 cups of water.
3. Garnish with beautiful lavender sprigs and ice!

Nutrition Facts: Calories: 248 | Carbohydrates: 65 g | Protein: 1 g | Fat: 1 g | Cholesterol: 172 mg

112. FROZEN LEMONADE WITH PINEAPPLE

Prep Time: 10 minutes
Cook Time: 10 minutes
Total Time: 20 minutes
Servings: 8

Ingredients:
- Six cups of frozen pineapple chunks
- 3/4 cup of fresh lemon juice (about 5 lemons)
- 1/2 cup of granulated sugar or equivalent alternative sweetener
- 2-4 cups of cold water
- 2-4 cups of ice

Directions:
1. 2 lemons, zested. Then, squeeze roughly 5 lemons to get 3/4 cup fresh juice.
2. In a blender, mix the lemon juice, lemon zest, sweetener of choice, and 2 cups water until completely blended.
3. In tiny increments, add frozen pineapple pieces, mixing thoroughly between additions.
4. 2 cups of ice should be added at the end. To get the required thickness, taste the mixture and add additional ice or water as needed. Serve right away.

Nutrition Facts: Calories: 308 | Carbohydrates: 80 g | Protein: 2 g | Fat: 0 g | Cholesterol: 73 mg

113. CUCUMBER ROSE APEROL SPRITZ

Prep Time: 5 minutes
Cook Time: 5 minutes
Total Time: 10 minutes
Servings: 1

Ingredients:
- oz rose-infused Aperol*
- 2 oz sparkling wine such as Prosecco
- 2 slices cucumber about an inch thick
- Splash club soda

Directions:
1. To make rose-infused Aperol, mix one 750ml bottle Aperol with one ounce dried rose petals (these can be found in the bulk section of most specialty food stores). Shake everything together and set it aside for a few hours or overnight. After straining off the rose petals, the Aperol is ready to use.
2. In a cocktail shaker, combine the Rose Aperol and cucumber with ice. Fill a tall Collins glass halfway with ice and strain it into it. Pour in the sparkling wine and ice. Garnish with fresh cucumber and a dash of club soda.

Nutrition Facts: Calories: 133 | Carbohydrates: 12 g | Protein: 2 g | Fat: 2 g | Cholesterol: 86 mg

114. THE BEST MARGARITA RECIPE

Prep Time: 10 minutes
Cook Time: 10 minutes
Total Time: 20 minutes
Servings: 10

Ingredients:
- 18 oz Tequila Blanco
- 18 oz fresh lime juice (fresh bottled lime juice from the refrigerated area, but not concentrated lime juice) FRESH)
- 9 oz. La Belle or Grand Marnier liqueur
- 8 oz simple syrup + a little more for the rims of the glasses
- 3 oz Triple Sec
- 3 oz orange juice
- Coarse or flake sea salt for the rims of the glasses
- Lime and orange slices for garnish

Directions:

1. If you don't have any on hand, start by preparing some simple syrup. 7 oz sugar and 7 oz water Microwave until the sugar is completely dissolved. You should have around 9-10 oz left over for rimming the glasses.
2. Combine all of the margarita ingredients in a big pitcher. Chill after thoroughly stirring.
3. Pour the simple leftover syrup into a shallow dish when ready to serve. In a second shallow dish, add sea salt (or flake salt). Then, dip the rims of the glasses in simple syrup, followed by salt.
4. If preferred, add ice to the glasses, and fill a shaker halfway with ice. Shake the margarita mix for 10-15 seconds in a shaker. Pour into serving glasses. Serve the cups garnished with cut limes or oranges. Ole'!

Nutrition Facts: Calories: 300 | Carbohydrates: 32 g | Protein: 0 g | Fat: 0 g | Cholesterol: 98 mg

115. SPICY PINEAPPLE HABANERO MARGARITAS

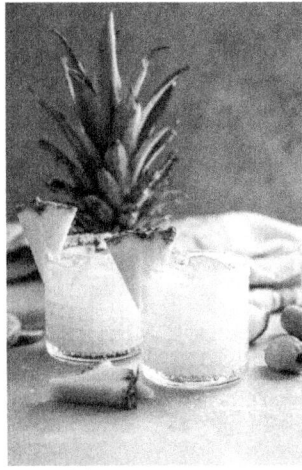

Prep Time: 5 minutes
Cook Time: 5 minutes
Total Time: 10 minutes
Servings: 6

Ingredients:
- 1 cup tequila silver
- 1 cup triple sec
- 1 cup fresh-squeezed lime juice
- 2 1/2 cups pineapple juice
- 4 habanero chiles
- Optional garnishes: salt, limes, habaneros, pineapple slices

Directions:
1. Melt the butter in a small pan over medium heat. Remove the seeds from the habaneros by cutting them in half. Place the chiles in the skillet and cook until they are blistered on both sides. Remove from the heat.
2. In a pitcher, combine the tequila, triple sec, lime juice, and pineapple juice. Stir everything together thoroughly.
3. Toss in the blistered habaneros. Allow them to soak in the margarita mix for 15 minutes to overnight. The longer they soak in the mixture, the hotter it will get. After 15 minutes, taste the mixture to see how long you want to soak them. When the heat level is to your taste, remove the habaneros.
4. Pour the margaritas into glasses with ice when ready to serve. Garnish with lime wedges, pineapple slices, or more habaneros if desired.

Nutrition Facts: Calories: 287 | Carbohydrates: 31 g | Protein: 1 g | Fat: 0 g | Cholesterol: 283 mg

116. WHOLEMEAL SODA BREAD

Prep Time: 10 minutes
Cook Time: 25 minutes
Total Time: 35 minutes
Servings: 4

Ingredients:
- 450g wholemeal flour, plus extra for dusting
- 75g four- mix (sunflower, golden lin and pumpkin)

- 2 tablespoon bicarbonate of soda
- 4 tablespoon black treacle
- 150ml pot natural bio yogurt made up to 450ml with water

Directions:
1. Preheat the oven to 200°C/180°C fan/gas 6 and line a baking sheet with parchment paper. In a large mixing basin, combine the flour, s, bicarbonate of soda, and a pinch of salt. When the treacle has dissolved in the yogurt mixture, pour it over the dry ingredients. Stir everything together with a knife until you have a moist, sticky dough. Allow for 5 minutes (this allows time for the liquid to absorb into the bran).
2. Form the dough into a circle approximately 18cm wide on a lightly floured board. It will still be extremely sticky, so don't overwork it; treat it more like scone dough than bread dough. Bake for 25-30 minutes, or until the crust is brown and the loaf sounds hollow when tapped beneath.

Nutrition Facts: Calories: 183 | Carbohydrates: 27 g | Protein: 71 g | Fat: 3 g | Cholesterol: 162 mg

117. STRAWBERRY MARGARITA RECIPE

Prep Time: 10 minutes
Cook Time: 0 minutes
Total Time: 10 minutes
Servings: 4

Ingredients:
- 1 pound fresh strawberries, trimmed
- 1 cup tequila
- 3/4 cup fresh lime juice
- 2/3 cup strawberry jam
- 1/4 cup triple sec
- 10 mint leaves
- 3-4 cups ice
- Optional Garnish: margarita salt, lime slices, extra strawberries

Directions:
1. Prepare a big blender. Add the fresh-cut strawberries, tequila, lime juice, strawberry jam, triple sec, mint leaves, and ice to the container.
2. Blend until smooth.
3. Toppings: Paint additional strawberry jam around the rims of four glasses using a pastry brush. Dip the rims of the glasses in margarita salt.
4. Fill the glass halfway with cold margaritas. Serve with a fresh lime slice and a strawberry on top.

Nutrition Facts: Calories: 391 | Carbohydrates: 57 g | Protein: 1 g | Fat: 1 g | Cholesterol: 144 mg

118. CRANBERRY POMEGRANATE MARGARITA WITH SPICED RIM

Prep Time: 5 minutes
Cook Time: 5 minutes
Total Time: 10 minutes
Servings: 4

Ingredients:
- 2 cups cranberry pomegranate juice blend
- 2 cups tequila Blanco
- 1 cup fresh squeezed lime juice
- 1/2 cup triple sec
- 2 tablespoons coarse sea salt
- 1 teaspoon Old El Paso Taco Seasoning
- 2 tablespoons agave syrup

Directions:
1. 1 tablespoon water and 1 tablespoon agave syrup on a dish To combine, gently mix everything together.
2. On a separate dish, combine the salt and Old El Paso Taco Seasoning.
3. Using the agave syrup, coat the rims of 4-6 glasses. Then, dip the rims in the seasoned salt. Fill the cups halfway with ice.

4. In a large ice-filled shaker or pitcher, combine the cranberry pomegranate juice, tequila, lime juice, and triple sec. Shake or mix before pouring into glasses and serving!

Nutrition Facts: Calories: 483 | Carbohydrates: 12 g | Protein: 2 g | Fat: 2 g | Cholesterol: 86 mg

119. HABANERO MARGARITAS

Prep Time: 5 minutes
Cook Time: 5 minutes
Total Time: 10 minutes
Servings: 6

Ingredients:
- 1 cup tequila silver
- 1 cup triple sec
- 1 cup fresh-squeezed lime juice
- Two and a half cups pineapple juice
- 4 habanero chiles
- Optional garnishes: salt, limes, habaneros, pineapple slices

Directions:
1. In a small saucepan over medium heat, melt the butter. Remove the seeds from the habaneros by cutting them in half. Place the chiles in the skillet and cook until they are blistered on both sides. Remove from the heat.
2. In a pitcher, combine the tequila, triple sec, lime juice, and pineapple juice. Stir everything together thoroughly.
3. Toss in the blistered habaneros. Allow them to soak in the margarita mix for 15 minutes to overnight. The longer they soak in the mixture, the hotter it will get. After 15 minutes, taste the mixture to see how long you want to soak them. When the heat level is to your taste, remove the habaneros.
4. Pour the margaritas into glasses with ice when ready to serve. Garnish with lime wedges, pineapple slices, or more habaneros if desired.

Nutrition Facts: Calories: 287 | Carbohydrates: 31 g | Protein: 1 g | Fat: 0 g | Cholesterol: 0 mg

120. BAHAMIAN BLASTER PARTY PUNCH RECIPE

Prep Time: 5 minutes
Cook Time: 5 minutes
Total Time: 10 minutes
Servings: 32

Ingredients:
- Quarts pineapple-orange juice (7 1/2 cups)
- 1.8 quarts pink grapefruit juice (7 1/2 cups)
- Three cups of gold rum
- Three cups of coconut rum
- Three cups of mango rum
- Three cups of passion fruit rum
- Three cups of pineapple rum
- One cup of banana rum (or banana liqueur)
- 3/4 cup grenadine

Directions:
1. Refrigerate all ingredients in a big 2-gallon jug or beverage dispenser until ready to serve.
2. If desired, garnish with fresh fruit.

Nutrition Facts: Calories: 318 | Carbohydrates: 19 g | Protein: 1 g | Fat: 1 g | Cholesterol: 110 mg

121. CHAMPAGNE HOLIDAY PUNCH RECIPE

Prep Time: 2 minutes
Cook Time: 2 minutes
Total Time: 4 minutes
Servings: 16

Ingredients:
- 750 ml of champagne (1 bottle)
- 24 oz of ginger beer (2 bottles)

- Three cups of cranberry juice cocktail (or juice blend)
- Two cups of ruby red grapefruit juice
- One cup of spiced rum, optional
- Possible Garnishes: fresh cranberries, grapefruit slices, cinnamon sticks

Directions:
1. All ingredients should be chilled. When ready to serve, combine all of the ingredients in a punch bowl.
2. Serve with cranberries, grapefruit slices, and cinnamon sticks as garnish.

Nutrition Facts: Calories: 108 | Carbohydrates: 13 g | Protein: 0 g | Fat: - g | Cholesterol: 7 mg

122. PERFECT MANHATTAN RECIPE

Prep Time: 2 minutes
Cook Time: 5 minutes
Total Time: 7 minutes
Servings: 1

Ingredients:
- 2 oz bourbon or rye whiskey
- 1-ounce sweet vermouth like Antica
- 2 dashes of angostura bitters
- Garnishes: twist of lemon rind, orange rind, or a maraschino cherry

Directions:
1. Fill a cocktail shaker halfway with ice for each Manhattan Cocktail. Combine the bourbon, sweet vermouth, and bitters in a mixing glass.
2. Using a bar spoon, stir everything together. Don't jiggle. Then strain into a coupe cocktail glass or a low ball glass filled with ice.
3. Serve with a maraschino cherry, lemon peel twist, or orange rind twist as a garnish.

Nutrition Facts: Calories: 190 | Carbohydrates: 2 g | Protein: 1 g | Fat: 1 g | Cholesterol: 9 mg

123. CHOCOLATE GUINNESS FLOAT RECIPE

Prep Time: 2 minutes
Cook Time: 5 minutes
Total Time: 7 minutes
Servings: 1

Ingredients:
- 2 scoops of chocolate ice cream
- 12 ounce Guinness beer

Directions:
1. In a tall glass, place 2 big scoops of chocolate ice cream.
2. Pour the Guinness over the top and serve immediately!

Nutrition Facts: Calories: 286 | Carbohydrates: 37 g | Protein: 5 g | Fat: 15 g | Cholesterol: 33 mg

124. BERRY BLAST NIMBU PANI

Prep Time: 10 minutes
Cook Time: 5 minutes
Total Time: 15 minutes
Servings: 4

Ingredients:
- 1 1/2 cup water
- 1 1/2 cup sugar
- 1 3/4 teaspoons salt
- 6 cups water or seltzer water
- 6 juicy limes
- 1 cup fresh strawberries or blackberries

Directions:
1. Combine one and half cups water, sugar, and salt in a small pot. Heat the sugar and salt until they melt into a sweet and salty simple syrup over medium-high heat. Place in the refrigerator to chill. Makes little more than 2 cups.
2. In the bottom of a pitcher, muddle (smash to smithereens) the berries.
3. Pour the lime juice into a pitcher and top with the simple cooled syrup. Stir in the additional water of seltzer water.

Nutrition Facts: Calories: 332 | Carbohydrates: 88 g | Protein: 1 g | Fat: 1 g | Cholesterol: 50 mg

125. SALMON GRILLED WITH SWEET AND SOUR PINEAPPLE SALSA

Prep Time: 10 minutes
Cook Time: 7 minutes
Total Time: 17 minutes
Servings: 6

Ingredients:
- 1 whole wild-caught salmon fillet (1.5-2 pounds)
- 1 tablespoon Tastefully Simple® Avocado Oil
- 3 teaspoons Tastefully Simple® Seasoning Salt, divided
- ¾ cup Tastefully Simple® Sweet & Sour Pineapple Sauce, divided
- 2 cups fresh pineapple, diced
- ½ cup diced red onion
- ¼ cup fresh chopped cilantro
- 1 whole jalapeno, shaved
- 2 cloves garlic, minced

Directions:
1. Preheat the grill to medium (350-400 degrees F).
2. Place the salmon fillet on a large baking sheet lined with foil. Pat the salmon dry with a paper towel and set it aside to dry for a few minutes while you prepare the salsa.
3. Cut up all of the fresh vegetables. Combine the pineapple, onion, cilantro, jalapeño, and garlic in a medium mixing bowl. 14 cup TS Sweet & Sour Pineapple Sauce and 1 teaspoon TS Seasoning Salt To mix, stir everything together.
4. 1 tablespoon avocado oil should be poured over the salmon fillet. Brush the oil over the fillet's surface. Then, on top of the salmon, sprinkle with 1-2 tablespoons TS Seasoning Salt.
5. Flip the salmon, skin-side up, onto the grill. 2 minutes on the grill Then, using two big spatulas, turn the salmon skin-side down. Brush the salmon with 12 cup TS Sweet & Sour Pineapple Sauce and cook for additional 5-8 minutes. When touched, the thickest end of the salmon should bounce back (rather than being mushy), but it should still be tender.
6. Remove the foil. Return the entire salmon fillet to the baking sheet with two big spatulas.
7. Serve the salsa on top of the salmon fillets while still warm.

Nutrition Facts: Calories: 290 | Carbohydrates: 26 g | Protein: 24 g | Fat: 10 g | Cholesterol: 72 mg

126. AHI TUNA BURGERS WITH GRILLED PINEAPPLE

Prep Time: 20 minutes
Cook Time: 10 minutes
Total Time: 30 minutes
Servings: 6

Ingredients:
For the Ahi Tuna Patties
- 2 pounds ahi tuna steaks diced
- 3 tablespoons soy sauce
- 1/4 cup light mayonnaise
- 1 tablespoon Sriracha chili sauce
- 1 large egg
- 1 cup chopped scallions, greens, and whites
- 1 tablespoon fresh grated ginger
- 2 tablespoons sesame
- 3/4 cup panko bread crumbs
- Sesame oil for cooking

For the Hoisin Mustard
- 1/4 cup Dijon mustard
- 1/4 cup hoisin sauce
- 1 tablespoon honey or sugar

For the Tuna Burgers
- 6 hamburger buns
- 6 slices fresh pineapple, round

- 1 ripe avocado sliced
- 6 leaves butter lettuce

Directions:
1. In a large mixing bowl, combine all of the ingredients for the ahi tuna patties. Divide the mixture into 6 equal pieces and shape it into patties. Preheat a griddle (or a skillet) over medium heat. When the surface is extremely hot, rub it with sesame oil and lay the patties on it. Sear the patties for 3 minutes per side, or until the inner ahi pieces are pink. Flip with caution. These patties are delicate.
2. The pineapple slices should then be grilled or seared for 1-2 minutes on each side.
3. To make the hoisin mustard, combine all of the ingredients in a mixing bowl. Then, put the mustard on the buns and pile on the lettuce, ahi tuna patties, grilled pineapple, and fresh avocado slices. Serve hot!

Nutrition Facts: Calories: 570 | Carbohydrates: 53 g | Protein: 45 g | Fat: 19 g | Cholesterol: 128 mg

127. **LEMONADE FUDGE**

Prep Time: 5 minutes
Cook Time: 5 minutes
Total Time: 10 minutes
Servings: 39

Ingredients:
- 20-ounce vanilla almond bark
- 14 ounce sweetened condensed milk
- 1 teaspoon lemon extract
- 2/3 cup chopped freeze-dried strawberries

Directions:
1. In a large microwave-safe bowl, place the sweetened condensed milk. Place the almond bark in a basin and roughly chop it. Microwave the mixture in 1-minute intervals, stirring in between, until completely smooth. (It takes around 2 minutes.)
2. Line an 8x8-inch baking dish with foil in the meanwhile. When the fudge mixture is smooth, add the lemon essence and strawberries. If desired, add yellow food coloring.
3. Place the fudge in the prepared pan and refrigerate for at least one hour. Then, transfer the firm fudge to a cutting board and peel off the foil. Trim the edges and cut the fabric into 49 squares. Keep at room temperature in an airtight container.

Nutrition Facts: Calories: 105 | Carbohydrates: 16 g | Protein: 1 g | Fat: 4 g | Cholesterol: 76 mg

128. **PINK LEMONADE CUPCAKES**

Prep Time: 30 minutes
Cook Time: 20 minutes
Total Time: 50 minutes
Servings: 24

Ingredients:
For the Pink Lemonade Cupcakes
- 3/4 cup Land O Lakes® Salted Butter softened (3 Half Sticks)
- 1 1/2 cups granulated sugar
- 2 large eggs
- 1 tablespoon vanilla extract
- 2 1/2 teaspoons baking powder
- 4 Meyer lemons 2 heaping tablespoons zest + 1/2 cup juice
- 2 1/2 cups all-purpose flour
- 3/4 cup whole milk
- 3 to 5 drops red food coloring

For the Pink Lemonade Frosting
- 1 1/2 cups Land O Lakes® Salted Butter softened (6 Half Sticks)
- 8 oz cream cheese softened
- 6-8 cups powdered sugar
- 1 Meyer lemon zest + 3 tablespoons juice
- 2 -3 drops red food coloring
- Pink Sprinkles
- 24 lemon jelly candy wedges

Directions:

1. Preheat the oven to 350 degrees Fahrenheit. Line two large muffin tins with paper liners (24 total). In the bowl of an electric mixer, combine 3 softened Land O Lakes® Salted Butter Half Sticks. Add the sugar and beat for 3 to 4 minutes, or until light and fluffy. Scrape down the sides of the basin and stir in the eggs, vanilla essence, and baking powder. To mix, beat the ingredients together.
2. To the bowl, add the lemon zest and juice. Reduce the mixer speed to low and gradually add the flour and milk until barely incorporated. Scrape the bowl once more and set the mixer on low while adding 3 to 5 drops of red food coloring to make a faint pink hue.
3. Distribute the batter equally among 24 cupcake liners. Bake for 15–20 minutes, or until a toothpick inserted into a cupcake comes out clean. Cool for 10 minutes in the muffin molds before transferring to a cooling rack.
4. Make the icing once the cupcakes have totally cooled. In a separate dish, combine the softened butter and cream cheese. At high speed, cream the mixture until it is very smooth and free of clumps. Scrape down the sides of the bowl, then add the lemon zest and juice. Turn the mixer to low and gradually add the powdered sugar until you achieve the desired consistency. To make a pale pink color, add 2 to 3 drops of red food coloring.
5. Fill a big piping bag with frosting and a wide pipe tip. Large mounds of frosting should be piped on top of each cupcake. Then top with pink sprinkles and a lemon jelly candy.

Nutrition Facts: Calories: 396 | Carbohydrates: 54 g | Protein: 3 g | Fat: 19 g | Cholesterol: 43 mg

129. SALTY DOG COCKTAIL RECIPE

Prep Time: 3 minutes
Cook Time: 3 minutes
Total Time: 6 minutes
Servings: 1

Ingredients:
- Four oz ruby red grapefruit juice
- Two oz vodka
- One ounce of club soda or sparkling grapefruit-flavored water
- 1-2 teaspoons of simple syrup
- Ice
- For Garnish: Kosher salt or Fleur de Sel agave syrup, grapefruit wedges

Directions:
1. Set out two tiny shallow plates for the Salt Rim. In one plate, spread salt, and in the other, spread a thin layer of agave syrup (or just syrup). Dip the edge of a highball glass in the syrup before dipping it in the salt.
2. Fill the glass three-quarters full of ice for each cocktail. Combine the grapefruit juice, vodka, club soda, and 1 teaspoon simple syrup in a mixing bowl.
3. Use a cocktail swizzle stick to stir. If desired, add a bit extra simple syrup to taste. Serve with a fresh grapefruit slice on the rim.

Nutrition Facts: Calories: 202 | Carbohydrates: 18 g | Protein: 1 g | Fat: 1 g | Cholesterol: 16 mg

130. GRAPEFRUIT SPARKLER

Prep Time: 5 minutes
Cook Time: 5 minutes
Total Time: 10 minutes
Servings: 1

Ingredients:
- 1 1/2 oz London dry style gin
- 3/4 ounce grapefruit cordial see recipe below

- 5 or 6 fresh mint leaves
- Prosecco or another sparkling wine

Directions:

To make Grapefruit Cordial
1. In a mixing dish, combine one cup of granulated sugar. 2 grapefruits, zest with a Microplane over sugar. Allow it to rest for at least an hour after thoroughly incorporating the zest and sugar (up to overnight). Juice the two grapefruits that were previously used and add them into the sugar/zest mixture. The sugar should melt quickly. Remove any solids and bottle.

To make the Grapefruit Sparkler
1. Shake the gin, cordial, and mint leaves vigorously together over ice. Top with sparkling wine and strain into a chilled cocktail glass.

Nutrition Facts: Calories: 116 | Carbohydrates: 4 g | Protein: 1 g | Fat: 1 g | Cholesterol: 63 mg

131. GRAPEFRUIT BASIL SORBET

Prep Time: 35 minutes
Cook Time: 20 minutes
Total Time: 55 minutes
Servings: 6

Ingredients:
- Four large of ruby red grapefruits, juiced
- Two cups of water
- One 3/4 cups of organic cane sugar or palm sugar
- Two lemons, zested and juiced
- One cup of basil leaves, packed
- pinch salt

Directions:
1. In a small saucepan, bring the water and sugar to a boil. When the water is boiling, add the lemon zest, basil leaves, and salt. Remove from the heat and cover with a lid. For at least 20 minutes, steep the basil leaves in the simple syrup.
2. Meanwhile, fill a 4-cup measuring pitcher halfway with lemon juice. Juice the grapefruits into the pitcher until 3 glasses of combined juices are measured.
3. Remove the basil leaves and strain the simple syrup. Then combine the syrup and the juice. Refrigerate for at least 2-3 hours (or to speed up, put in the freezer for 1 hour.)
4. Fill an electric ice cream maker halfway with the sorbet mixture. Turn on and mix for at least 20 minutes, or until the mixture achieves a "soft-serve" consistency.
5. Sorbet may be eaten right away or frozen in an airtight container. Allow the sorbet to soften for 10-15 minutes after it has been frozen before serving.

Nutrition Facts: Calories: 272 | Carbohydrates: 70 g | Protein: 1 g | Fat: 1 g | Cholesterol: 68 mg

132. PINK GRAPEFRUIT MARGARITA

Prep Time: 5 minutes
Cook Time: 5 minutes
Total Time: 10 minutes
Servings: 2

Ingredients:
- Five oz of freshly squeezed ruby red grapefruit juice
- Four oz white tequila
- 1 1/2 oz Triple Sec orange liquor
- 1/2 ounce agave syrup + extra for glass rims
- Fresh grapefruit slices for garnish
- Salt for rim

Directions:
1. Put a little quantity of agave syrup on one plate and salt on another. Dip the rims of the glasses first in the syrup, then in the salt. Fill the cups halfway with ice and set them aside.

2. Fill an ice-filled cocktail shaker halfway with ice. Fill the shaker halfway with fresh grapefruit juice, tequila, Triple Sec, and agave.
3. Cover and vigorously shake for 30 seconds. After that, pour into the glasses. Enjoy with fresh grapefruit slices as a garnish!

Nutrition Facts: Calories: 251 | Carbohydrates: 20 g | Protein: 1 g | Fat: 1 g | Cholesterol: 115 mg

133. BRULEED GRAPEFRUIT (PAMPLEMOUSSE BRÛLÉ)

Prep Time: 5 minutes
Cook Time: 8 minutes
Total Time: 13 minutes
Servings: 8

Ingredients:
- Four large ripe ruby red grapefruits
- Eight teaspoons granulated sugar
- Brulee Torch

Directions:
1. Cup your hand around the top of a grapefruit stem from top to bottom, starting with your index finger. Then, cut it in half straight down the middle. (If you don't notice a floral pattern, you've sliced the grapefruit incorrectly.) Each grapefruit should be cut in this manner.
2. Cut along the inside rim of each grapefruit half with a tiny serrated knife, removing the fruit from the peel. Then, using a spoon, cut along the membrane between each small triangle section so that each mouthful comes out easily. Keep everything as is.
3. Sprinkle 1 teaspoon granulated sugar over the top of each grapefruit half, one at a time. Then, with the flame held over the grapefruit, Brulee the top until the sugar becomes golden and the top of each half is candied. This should take between 30 and 60 seconds per half. Serve right away and then repeat.

Nutrition Facts: Calories: 67 | Carbohydrates: 12 g | Protein: 2 g | Fat: 2 g | Cholesterol: 86 mg

134. BEST MAI TAI COCKTAIL RECIPE

Prep Time: 5 minutes
Cook Time: 5 minutes
Total Time: 10 minutes
Servings: 1

Ingredients:
Mexican mai tai variation
- 1 1/2 oz reposado tequila
- 3/4 ounce fresh lime juice
- 1/2 ounce orange curacao I like to use Cointreau Noir
- 1/2 ounce orgeat
- 2 oz aged pot still rum (or blended rum)
- 3/4 ounce fresh lime juice
- 3/4 ounce Cointreau (or orange curacao)
- 1/3 ounce rich simple syrup (2:1 sugar to water ratio)
- 1/4 ounce orgeat
- Garnishes: mint, lime, pineapple, maraschino cherries

Directions:
1. Fill an 8-ounce shaker halfway with ice. Combine all of the ingredients. Cover and gently shake for 30 seconds.
2. Fill a tiki mug or low ball glass halfway with the contents (including the ice). The traditional Mai Tai garnishes are mint and lime. When served in tiki cups, though, pineapple and cherries are ideal.

Citrus salt

1. To create citrus salt, use a Microplane to grate the zest of an orange and lime. Stir the zest into the salt and let it aside for 10 minutes to enable the citrus oils to coat the salt.
2. Use the citrus salt to rim a rock's glass. Shake the tequila, lime, curacao, and orgeat with ice and pour into a salted glass over ice.

Nutrition Facts: Calories: 183 | Carbohydrates: 10 g | Protein: 1 g | Fat: 1 g | Cholesterol: 62 mg

2. For each drink, prepare Half-fill a glass with ice. Over ice, combine the simple syrup, lemon juice, and gin. Top with club soda after stirring.
3. To make a martini-style Tom Collins, use the following ingredients: Fill an ice-filled cocktail shaker halfway with ice. Combine the simple syrup, lemon, and gin in a mixing glass. Shake for 30-60 seconds, or until foamy. Add 1-2 oz of club soda to a martini glass.

Nutrition Facts: Calories: 213 | Carbohydrates: 21 g | Protein: 1 g | Fat: 1 g | Cholesterol: 62 mg

135. LAVENDER MEYER LEMON TOM COLLINS COCKTAIL

Prep Time: 30 minutes
Cook Time: 5 minutes
Total Time: 35 minutes
Servings: 1

Ingredients:
For the Simple Syrup
- 1 1/4 cup water
- 1 cup granulated sugar
- 1 bunch lavender buds, stems and leaves (or 3 tablespoons dried culinary buds)

For each Tom Collins Cocktail
- 1-ounce lavender simple syrup
- 1 ounce Meyer lemon juice about 1/2 a lemon
- 2 oz good gin
- Ice
- Club soda

Directions:
1. In a small saucepan over high heat, combine the water, sugar, and lavender. Bring to a gentle boil, then remove from heat and cover. Allow for a 20-minute steeping time for the simple syrup. To remove the lavender, strain the mixture through a strainer. Keep refrigerated until ready to use.

136. BRANDY JAVA ICE

Prep Time: 2 minutes
Cook Time: 2 minutes
Total Time: 4 minutes
Servings: 2

Ingredients:
- 4 scoops vanilla ice cream large
- 2 oz brandy
- 2 teaspoon ground coffee, not instant granules

Directions:
2. In a blender, combine all of the ingredients and puree until smooth. Enjoy!

Nutrition Facts: Calories: 339 | Carbohydrates: 21 g | Protein: 5 g | Fat: 15 g | Cholesterol: 100 mg

137. LAVENDER MEYER LEMON TOM COLLINS COCKTAIL

Prep Time: 30 minutes
Cook Time: 5 minutes
Total Time: 35 minutes
Servings: 1

Ingredients:

For the Simple Syrup
- 1 1/4 cup water
- 1 cup granulated sugar
- 1 bunch lavender buds, stems and leaves (or 3 tablespoons dried culinary buds)

For each Tom Collins Cocktail
- One ounce simple lavender syrup
- One ounce Meyer lemon juice about 1/2 a lemon
- Two oz good gin
- Ice
- Club soda

Directions:
1. In a small saucepan over high heat, combine the water, sugar, and lavender. Bring to a gentle boil, then remove from heat and cover. Allow for a 20-minute steeping time for the simple syrup. To remove the lavender, strain the mixture through a strainer. Keep refrigerated until ready to use.
2. For each drink, prepare Half-fill a glass with ice. Over ice, combine the simple syrup, lemon juice, and gin. Top with club soda after stirring.
3. To make a martini-style Tom Collins, use the following ingredients: Fill an ice-filled cocktail shaker halfway with ice. Combine the simple syrup, lemon, and gin in a mixing glass. Shake for 30-60 seconds, or until foamy. Add 1-2 oz of club soda to a martini glass.

Nutrition Facts: Calories: 213 | Carbohydrates: 21 g | Protein: 1 g | Fat: 1 g | Cholesterol: 17 mg

138. <u>WINE PUNCH COCKTAILS</u>

Prep Time: 5 minutes
Cook Time: 5 minutes
Total Time: 10 minutes
Servings: 24

Ingredients:
- liters red wine (I used a boxed California blend)
- 4 cups cranberry-apple juice
- 3 cups orange juice
- 36 oz ginger beer or strong ginger soda
- 5 teaspoons vanilla extract

Possible Garnishes
- fresh cranberries, orange slices, apple slices, fresh mint, cinnamon sticks

Directions:
1. In a large punch bowl, combine the red wine, both juices, ginger beer, and vanilla extract. To combine, stir everything together thoroughly.
2. Garnish with fresh fruit and cinnamon sticks, if desired. Serve with ice.

Nutrition Facts: Calories: 102 | Carbohydrates: 13 g | Protein: 0 g | Fat: 0 g | Cholesterol: 63 mg

139. <u>BLASTER PARTY PUNCH RECIPE</u>

Prep Time: 5 minutes
Cook Time: 5 minutes
Total Time: 10 minutes
Servings: 32

Ingredients:
- quarts pineapple-orange juice (7 1/2 cups)
- 1.8 quarts pink grapefruit juice (7 1/2 cups)
- 3 cups gold rum
- 3 cups coconut rum
- 3 cups mango rum
- 3 cups passion fruit rum
- 2 cups pineapple rum
- 1 cup banana rum (or banana liqueur)
- 3/4 cup grenadine

Directions:
1. Refrigerate all ingredients in a big 2-gallon jug or beverage dispenser until ready to serve.
2. If desired, garnish with fresh fruit.

Notes: This recipe yields 2 gallons of party punch or 32 8-ounce drinks.

Nutrition Facts: Calories: 318 | Carbohydrates: 19 g | Protein: 1 g | Fat: 1 g | Cholesterol: 195 mg

140. SMASH CARIBBEAN COCKTAILS

Prep Time: 5 minutes
Cook Time: 3 minutes
Total Time: 8 minutes
Servings: 40

Ingredients:
- 14 cups 100% pineapple juice
- 2 bottles of dark Caribbean rum (750 ml each - I used Pusser's)
- 1 bottle coconut rum (750 ml - Cruzan)
- 2 cups fresh-squeezed lime juice
- 1 1/2 cups simple syrup
- 1 cup orange liqueur (Cointreau)
- 1/2 teaspoon bitters, optional
- Fresh pineapple slices for garnish

Directions:
1. If you're creating your own simple syrup, mix 1 cup granulated sugar and 1 cup water. Cook until the sugar melts on the burner. Allow cooling fully.
2. Fill a big beverage dispenser halfway with all of the ingredients. Stir everything together thoroughly. Chill until ready to serve, then top with cut pineapples.
3. Serve with ice.

Nutrition Facts: Calories: 222 | Carbohydrates: 16 g | Protein: 1 g | Fat: 1 g | Cholesterol: 118 mg

141. CRANBERRY SMOOTHIE

Prep Time: 5 minutes
Cook Time: 0 minutes
Total Time: 5 minutes
Servings: 1

Ingredients:
- 75g / ¾ cup of frozen cranberries (or fresh cranberries but add a handful of ice too)
- One large apple cored and chopped into chunks
- One small handful / about Two tablespoons of raw pecans or walnuts (see notes for nut-free option)
- One tablespoon maple syrup
- 240mls / 1 cup non-dairy milk
- ¼ teaspoon ground cinnamon

Directions:
1. Add all the ingredients to a blender.
2. Blend until smooth.

Nutrition Facts: Calories: 424 | Carbohydrates: 61 g | Protein: 10 g | Fat: 19 g | Cholesterol: 251 mg

142. NO-WAIT FROSÉ RECIPE

Prep Time: 5 minutes
Cook Time: 5 minutes
Total Time: 10 minutes
Servings: 8

Ingredients:
- ½ cup vodka
- ½ cup granulated sugar
- 16 oz whole frozen strawberries
- 750 ml bottle rosé wine
- 1-3 cups ice cubes if needed

Directions:
1. Prepare a big, high-powered blender. Combine the vodka and sugar in a mixing bowl. To dissolve the sugar, cover and purée for 1 minute.
2. Then stir in the frozen strawberries and rosé. Puree till smooth, covered. Examine the consistency. To thicken the frosé, add 1-3 cups of ice as required. If necessary, puree once more. ** Depending on the strength of your blender, ice isn't always essential. In the summer, when the house is warm, I generally add around 2 cups of ice.

3. Serve immediately or place in the freezer until ready to use. Because of the alcohol component, the Frosé will not completely freeze through, but you may leave it in the freezer for many hours if necessary.

Nutrition Facts: Calories: 178 | Carbohydrates: 22 g | Protein: 1 g | Fat: 1 g | Cholesterol: 87 mg

5. Would you want to make a Virgin Bloody Mary? Simply leave out the vodka. When serving, you can add a dash of club soda or drink it as is.

Nutrition Facts: Calories: 154 | Carbohydrates: 14 g | Protein: 2 g | Fat: 2 g | Cholesterol: 408 mg

143. LT. DAN'S BEST BLOODY MARY MIX RECIPE (HOMEMADE!)

Prep Time: 5 minutes
Cook Time: 0 minutes
Total Time: 5 minutes
Servings: 4

Ingredients:
- 4 cups clamato (or tomato juice)
- 6 oz vodka
- 2 oz fresh lemon juice
- 1-ounce fresh lime juice
- 1 ½ tablespoon prepared horseradish
- 1 tablespoon Worcestershire sauce
- 1 teaspoon hot sauce (your favorite brand)
- ½ teaspoon garlic powder
- ½ teaspoon celery salt
- ½ teaspoon smoked paprika

Directions:
1. Prepare a big 6-8 cup pitcher. Combine the clamato, vodka, lemon juice, and lime juice in a mixing bowl. Stir.
2. Then measure and combine all of the remaining ingredients. Stir everything together thoroughly.
3. Refrigerate until ready to serve, covered. Fill cups halfway with ice and pour in the Bloody Mary mix.
4. Garnish with celery stalks, pickles, olives, pickled or raw veggies, lemon wedges, grilled shrimp, bacon, grilled or raw chiles, or anything else you like!

144. THAI COCONUT CURRY LENTIL SOUP

Prep Time: 15 minutes
Cook Time: 35 minutes
Total Time: 40 minutes
Servings: 4

Ingredients:
- 1 tablespoon olive oil
- 1 cup onion finely chopped
- 1 clove garlic minced
- 1 teaspoon ginger minced
- 1 teaspoon Thai red curry paste use 2 teaspoons if you like it spicy
- 6 cups low sodium vegetable broth
- 1 cup red lentils picked through for stones, rinsed
- One medium sweet potato cut into 1/2" pieces
- 1 stalk lemongrass tender bulb only, smashed with a mallet
- 2 kaffir lime leaves
- 1/4 teaspoon turmeric
- 1 teaspoon sea salt
- 1/4 cup coconut milk
- fresh kaffir lime leaf slivers or minced cilantro for garnish, optional

Directions:
1. In a medium saucepan, heat the olive oil. Then Combine the ginger, onions, and garlic in a mixing bowl. Cook for 3-4 minutes over medium heat or until softened.
2. Cook for several minutes or until the Thai red curry paste is aromatic.

3. Combine the broth, lentils, sweet potato, lemongrass, kaffir lime leaves, and turmeric in a mixing bowl. Bring to a boil, then lower to medium-low heat, cover, and simmer for 20-25 minutes, or until the lentils and sweet potatoes are tender.
4. Remove the lemongrass and kaffir lime leaves from the dish. Stir in the coconut milk and season with salt. Cook for another five minutes. If desired, puree.
5. Garnish with slivers of kaffir lime leaf or fresh cilantro and a drizzle of coconut milk.

Nutrition Facts: Calories: 312 | Carbohydrates: 12 g | Protein: 7 g | Fat: 49 g | Cholesterol: 15 mg

145. MINT JULEP (RECIPE)

Prep Time: 3 minutes
Cook Time: 3 minutes
Total Time: 6 minutes
Servings: 1

Ingredients:
- 5 – 6 fresh mint leaves
- 1/4 ounce concentrated simple syrup
- 2 oz high proof bourbon I prefer 4 Roses or Bulleit
- Shaved ice
- Mint leaf for garnish

Directions:
1. Fill copper glasses halfway with mint leaves and simple syrup. Muddle the simple syrup and mint lightly. (Do not crush the mint leaves; simply cover them with syrup and let the mint aroma mingle.)
2. Then add the bourbon and ice. Lightly whisk the ingredients into the ice with a bar spoon. Garnish with mint leaves on top.

Nutrition Facts: Calories: 159 | Carbohydrates: 7 g | Protein: 1 g | Fat: 1 g | Cholesterol: 182 mg

146. KILLER BEE COCKTAILS

Prep Time: 5 minutes
Cook Time: 5 minutes
Total Time: 10 minutes
Servings: 6

Ingredients:
- 2 cups of gold rum
- 2 cups of passionfruit juice
- 2 cups of freshly squeezed orange juice
- 1/4 cup of fresh lime juice
- ½ teaspoons of Wholesome® Organic Stevia
- 1/2 teaspoon of ground nutmeg
- Club Soda

Directions:
1. In a pitcher, combine the rum, passionfruit, orange, and lime juices.
2. Combine Wholesome® Organic Stevia, nutmeg in a mixing bowl. Stir until the stevia has completely dissolved into the beverage.
3. To be served: Fill glasses halfway with ice and pour the drink over them. Make a space at the top for the club soda. Add 2-3 teaspoons club soda to each glass. Add a fruity garnish and stir!

Notes: If you have time, refrigerate the mixture for at least 1 hour to enable the taste to develop.

Nutrition Facts: Calories: 249 | Carbohydrates: 16 g | Protein: 0 g | Fat: 0 g | Cholesterol: 52 mg

147. SPARKLING PINEAPPLE MINT JUICE

Prep Time: 10 minutes
Cook Time: 10 minutes
Total Time: 20 minutes
Servings: 2

Ingredients:
- Peeled and sliced fresh pineapple (save a few slices from garnishing if desired)

- Fresh mint, 1/4 cup (one tiny handful)
- A few tablespoons of honey or your preferred sweetness (optional)
- 1-liter sparkling water or club soda bottle
- To serve, crushed ice

Directions:
1. In a high-speed blender or food processor, combine the pineapple, mint, and sweetener (if using). Blend until smooth.
2. Fill tall glasses halfway with crushed ice. To finish, top with sparkling water or club soda.
3. Serve immediately, if desired, garnished with mint or pineapple pieces.

Nutrition Facts: Calories: 27 | Carbohydrates: 10 g | Protein: 2 g | Fat: 2 g | Cholesterol: 0 mg

148. SWEET TEA OLD FASHIONED COCKTAIL

Prep Time: 3 minutes
Cook Time: 3 minutes
Total Time: 6 minutes
Servings: 1

Ingredients:
- sugar cube
- dashes bitters
- lemon wedge or slice
- 1 orange wedge or slice
- 1-2 Maraschino cherries
- 1-ounce club soda
- 2 oz Fire Fly "Sweet Tea" vodka
- Ice

Directions:
1. Pour 2 dashes of bitters over the top of the sugar cube at the bottom of the glass. To dissolve the sugar cube, muddle.
2. Fill the glass halfway with ice, then squeeze in the lemon and orange wedges. Save the wedges for garnishing the glass.
3. Combine the club soda and Fire Fly Vodka in a mixing glass. Stir. Rub the lemon wedge over the rim of the glass, then garnish with the lemon wedge, orange wedge, and cherry.

Nutrition Facts: Calories: 234 | Carbohydrates: 19 g | Protein: 1 g | Fat: 1 g | Cholesterol: 62 mg

149. FROZEN BEERITAS RECIPE

Prep Time: 5 minutes
Cook Time: 5 minutes
Total Time: 10 minutes
Servings: 2

Ingredients:
- 3 oz tequila Blanco
- 1 oz Triple Sec (orange liqueur)
- 3 oz fresh lime juice
- 3 oz simple syrup
- 2 oz orange juice
- 1/4 oz Mexican beer, such as two 7-ounce Coronitas or one 12-ounce can of any Mexican beer
- 3-4 cups ice

Directions:
Self-Serve Method
1. In a blender, combine tequila, Triple Sec, lime juice, simple syrup, and orange juice. Pour with 3 glasses of ice. Puree the mixture until it is smooth and foamy. Serve the margaritas in two big tumblers, with a Coronita on the side. As they sip their Margarita, each individual can add beer to it.
2. In a blender, combine the tequila, Triple Sec, lime juice, simple syrup, orange juice, and a 12 ounce lager. Pour with 4 glasses of ice. Mash the mixture until it is smooth and foamy. Pour into serving glasses and serve.

Nutrition Facts: Calories: 386 | Carbohydrates: 51 g | Protein: 1 g | Fat: 0 g | Cholesterol: 55 mg

150. DECAF PEPPERMINT TEA

Prep Time: 5 minutes
Cook Time: 0 minutes
Total Time: 5 minutes
Servings: 1

Ingredients:
- 1 Teabag Peppermint Tea
- 8 oz water
- 2 tablespoon Artificial sweetener optional

Directions:
1. Fill a coffee cup halfway with teabags.
2. Place a teapot on the burner with the water. Wait for the whistle to blow. Pour it over the teabag.
3. -OR- Place the microwavable coffee cup in the microwave and heat for 30 seconds. Microwave for 2 minutes or until the desired temperature is reached.
4. Allow the tea to infuse for a few seconds in the water.
5. Stir in the artificial sweetener with a spoon until it dissolves. If the water is too hot for you, add an ice cube. Slurp, slurp, slurp!

Nutrition Facts: Calories: 220 | Carbohydrates: 12 g | Protein: 2 g | Fat: 2 g | Cholesterol: 86 mg

151. SUGAR-FREE ROOT BEER ICE POPS

Prep Time: 5 minutes
Cook Time: 180 minutes
Total Time: 185 minutes
Servings: 4

Ingredients:
- Packet Sugar-free on-the-go drink mix, like A&W Singles, To Drink Mix Root Beer Flavored
- 16 oz Water, bottled

Directions:
1. Pour the drink mix into a 16.9 fluid ounce bottle of water.
2. Twist the cap back on securely and shake to mix.
3. Pour four oz of liquid into each ice pop mold.
4. Insert the ice pop sticks with caution.
5. Freeze for three hours or until firm.

Nutrition Facts: Calories: 172 | Carbohydrates: 36 g | Protein: 28 g | Fat: 11 g | Cholesterol: 286 m

152. SYRUP (RECIPE)

Prep Time: 2 Minutes
Cook Time: 3 Minutes
Total Time: 5 Minutes
Servings: 8

Ingredients:
- 1 cup water
- 1 cup granulated sugar or turbinado, demerara

Directions:
1. Preheat a small saucepot to high. Fill the saucepan with water and sugar.
2. Bring to a boil, stirring constantly. Stir once the water has reached a boil, then remove from the heat. (Add the herbs to the simple heated syrup if you're infusing them.)
3. Allow cooling to room temperature before storing in an airtight container.

Nutrition Facts: Calories: 97 | Carbohydrates: 25 g | Protein: 25 g | Fat: 2 g | Cholesterol: 63 mg

CHAPTER 7: DINNER (CLEAR FLUIDS)

153. SWEET TEA

Prep Time: 3 minutes
Cook Time: 3 minutes
Total Time: 6 minutes
Servings: 8

Ingredients:
- 8 cups water
- 6 herbal tea bags
- 1/3 – 2/3 cup of sugar or sub your sweetener of choice

Directions:
1. Choose two varieties of herbal tea that you believe will complement each other. Fill a medium sauce saucepan halfway with water. Then, remove the paper tags from the tea bags and immerse them in water.
2. Once the water has reached a simmer, remove the heat and cover for 3-5 minutes to steep.
3. With a slotted spoon, remove the tea bags from the kettle and mix in the sugar. If you intend to serve the hot tea over ice right away, add additional sugar. Add less sugar if you intend to cool the concentrated tea before serving. In either case, serve chilled over ice.

Nutrition Facts: Calories: 97 | Carbohydrates: 25 g | Protein: 26 g | Fat: 11 g | Cholesterol: 26 mg

154. CANDIED ORANGE PEEL RECIPE

Prep Time: 35 minutes
Cook Time: 20 minutes
Total Time: 55 minutes
Servings: 20

Ingredients:
- 4 large navel oranges or 5 small
- 2 cups water
- ½ cups granulated sugar divided
- 2 teaspoon vanilla extract
- ½ teaspoon salt

Directions:
1. Trim the oranges' tops and bottoms. The oranges should next be peeled from top to bottom into 2-4 inch pieces using a vegetable peeler. To obtain a good uniform layer of peel, press the peeler firmly against the orange. The wide strips should next be cut into ¼ inch thin strips.
2. In a medium saucepot, combine the orange peel segments. Heat the oil over medium to medium-low heat. Combine the water, 1 cup of sugar, and salt in a mixing bowl. Bring to a boil. Set the timer for 20 minutes, or until the peels seem soft but keep their vivid color once boiling. (You don't want them to brown, so keep the stove just hot enough to keep the simmer going.)
3. Meanwhile, set aside the remaining 12 cups of sugar in a dish. Place a drying rack on the floor and cover it with wax or parchment paper.
4. Stir in the vanilla essence after the orange peels have simmered for 20 minutes. Turn off the heat and set aside the peels for 5 minutes in the sugar syrup.
5. To transfer the orange peels to the cooling rack, use tongs. Allow the orange peels to dry and cool for at least 15 minutes. Then, to coat, throw them in the sugar. Allow the peels to completely dry at room temperature. Then, place in an airtight container and refrigerate for up to 2 weeks.

Nutrition Facts: Calories: 71 | Carbohydrates: 18 g | Protein: 1 g | Fat: 1 g | Cholesterol: 59 mg

155. HOT BUTTERED RUM RECIPE

Prep Time: 5 minutes
Cook Time: 380 minutes

Total Time: 385 minutes
Servings: 16

Ingredients:
- 2 quarts water
- 2 cups light brown sugar packed
- ½ cup salted butter
- 4-6 cinnamon sticks
- 8-10 whole cloves
- 1 teaspoon ground nutmeg
- 1/8 teaspoon cayenne
- ½ cups spiced or dark rum
- 1/3 cup heavy cream

Directions:
1. In a large crock pot, combine the water, brown sugar, butter, and all spices. To dissolve the sugar, give it a good stir.
2. Cover the slow cooker and set it to HIGH for 3+ hours or LOW for 6+ hours.
3. Whisk in the rum and heavy cream when ready to serve. If necessary, season with salt or cayenne pepper. Pour into cups and serve hot.

Note: To prepare on the stovetop, mix all ingredients in a big saucepan, except the rum and heavy cream, and cook over medium-low heat. Bring to a moderate boil, stirring regularly, until the sugar dissolves. When ready to serve, remove from the heat and whisk in the rum and heavy cream.

Nutrition Facts: Calories: 262 | Carbohydrates: 28 g | Protein: 1 g | Fat: 5 g | Cholesterol: 22 mg

156. CARAMEL HOT APPLE CIDER RECIPE

Prep Time: 3 minutes
Cook Time: 10 minutes
Total Time: 13 minutes
Servings: 16

Ingredients:
- 1 gallon fresh apple cider
- 2 cup caramel flavored syrup as used in coffee drinks, such as Torani
- 1/2 - 1 tablespoons sea salt

Directions:
1. Warm the apple cider and caramel syrup in a big saucepan (or crock pot) to the appropriate temperature.
2. 1/2 teaspoon of sea salt Taste the Salted Caramel Apple Cider and adjust the sweetness as required.

Nutrition Facts: Calories: 162 | Carbohydrates: 40 g | Protein: 1 g | Fat: 1 g | Cholesterol: 245 mg

157. BONITA APPLE COCKTAIL (APPLE BUTTER RUM COCKTAILS)

Prep Time: 5 minutes
Cook Time: 5 minutes
Total Time: 10 minutes
Servings: 1

Ingredients:
For the Apple Butter Infused Aged Rum
- 750 ml bottle-aged rum We used Mount Gay Black Barrel
- 1 cup Musselman's Apple Butter

For the Bonita Apple Butter Cocktail
- 2 oz Apple Butter Infused Aged Rum
- 2 teaspoon Musselman's Apple Butter
- 1/2 teaspoon fresh lime juice
- 2 ounce fresh pineapple juice
- 1/4 ounce orange curacao Grand Marnier
- 1/2 ounce demerara sugar syrup 1:1 sugar to water
- ice
- Apple slices and lime wedges for garnish

Directions:
For the apple butter infused aged rum:
1. Allow the apple butter and aged rum to rest overnight. Then strain the liquid through a coffee filter.

For a Frozen Bonita Apple Butter Cocktail
1. Combine all of the ingredients in a blender with 1 1/2 cups ice. Blend until completely smooth. Then pour into a glass and garnish with a lemon twist.

For a Bonita Apple Butter Cocktail On the Rocks
1. In a cocktail shaker, combine all of the ingredients. Shake for 20 seconds with two handfuls of ice. Then, fill a glass halfway with ice and strain the cocktail into it. Garnish with parsley and serve.

Nutrition Facts: Calories: 211 | Carbohydrates: 18 g | Protein: 10 g | Fat: 19 g | Cholesterol: 37 mg

158. HOT APPLE CIDER WASSAIL RECIPE

Prep Time: 5 minutes
Cook Time: 260 minutes
Total Time: 265 minutes
Servings: 12

Ingredients:
- 1gallon Musselman's Apple Cider
- Four cups orange juice
- Four hibiscus tea bags
- Ten cinnamon sticks
- One teaspoon of whole cloves
- 2 tablespoon juniper berries
- ½ inch fresh ginger piece, cut into slices
- 1 apple, sliced into rounds
- 1 orange, sliced into rounds

Directions:
1. Cover and place all of the ingredients in a slow cooker.
2. Heat the slow cooker on high for 3-4 hours, or until the color has darkened and the fruit is tender. Remove the tea bags and serve immediately.

Nutrition Facts: Calories: 207 | Carbohydrates: 50 g | Protein: 14 g | Fat: 0 g | Cholesterol: 47 mg

159. MANGO SMOOTHIE

Prep Time: 10 minutes
Cook Time: 10 minutes
Total Time: 20 minutes
Servings: 4

Ingredients:
- Two ripe mangoes or Two cups of frozen mango
- cup boiling water
- 1 green tea bag
- cups ice
- ½ frozen banana
- honey optional

Directions:
1. Store the tea bags in the boiling water, then place them in the freezer to chill while you finish the smoothie.
2. Remove the pit from the mangoes and place the flesh in the blender. If desired, add the ice, half a frozen banana, and 1 tablespoon of honey.
3. Then, take the tea out of the freezer and throw away the tea bags. Fill the blender halfway with tea, cover, and puree until smooth. Serve right away.

Nutrition Facts: Calories: 63 | Carbohydrates: 16 g | Protein: 1 g | Fat: 1 g | Cholesterol: 214 mg

160. AUTHENTIC CHAI TEA RECIPE

Prep Time: 1 minute
Cook Time: 8 minutes
Total Time: 9 minutes
Servings: 4

Ingredients:
- Four cups water
- 1 whole star anise
- Two sticks of cinnamon
- Four cardamom pods, cracked
- 4-5 black tea bags, or 1/4 cup loose black tea
- 1 cups half & half, or whole milk
- 1/4 cup granulated sugar

Directions:

1. It's best to squeeze cardamom pods until they break. In a small saucepan, bring the water, tea, star anise, cinnamon, and cardamom to a boil.
2. Boil for 8-10 minutes, or until the tea has become black and reduced to approximately 2 cups. After straining, add the sugar. Stir in the half-and-half until it's hot.
3. For good friends, put the used cardamom pods in the bottom of the cups.

Nutrition Facts: Calories: 132 | Carbohydrates: 21 g | Protein: 12 g | Fat: 4 g | Cholesterol: 62 mg

161. JUGO VERDE (GREEN JUICE)

Prep Time: 10 minutes
Cook Time: 10 minutes
Total Time: 20 minutes
Servings: 5

Ingredients:
- 2 cups orange juice
- 1/2 cups fresh pineapple chunks
- 1/2 Nopal cactus paddle chopped (or substitute 1 celery stalk)
- large cucumber with peel, cut into chunks
- 1/4 cup packed parsley or cilantro

Directions:
1. In a blender, combine all of the ingredients. Add a bit of salt, close the lid tightly, and puree until smooth.
2. When the mixture is green and frothy, serve immediately or strain over a screen to remove the pulp.

Nutrition Facts: Calories: 78 | Carbohydrates: 18 g | Protein: 26 g | Fat: 19 g | Cholesterol: 63 mg

162. ASIAN BLOODY MARY COCKTAIL

Prep Time: 2 minutes
Cook Time: 2 minutes
Total Time: 4 minutes
Servings: 1

Ingredients:
- 5 oz tomato juice
- 1/2 teaspoon fish sauce
- 1/2 teaspoon soy sauce
- 1/2 teaspoon of chili garlic sauce or Sriracha
- 1/8 teaspoon wasabi paste
- 2 oz vodka
- 1/4 teaspoon
- 2-3 dashes of celery salt

Directions:
1. Combine all of the ingredients. Stir everything together thoroughly.
2. Check for heat and add more chili garlic sauce if necessary.
3. Pour over ice in a tall glass and garnish with a scallion or lemongrass sprig.

Nutrition Facts: Calories: 161 | Carbohydrates: 7 g | Protein: 2 g | Fat: 1 g | Cholesterol: 25 mg

163. AGUA FRESCA

Prep Time: 5 minutes
Cook Time: 5 minutes
Total Time: 10 minutes
Servings: 4

Ingredients:
- 2 cups fresh strawberries cold, hulled
- 2 cups fresh chopped pineapple cold
- 1 cup sugar
- 8 cups water cold

Directions:
1. In a blender, combine the chilled fruit, sugar, and water. Puree the mixture until it is smooth and foamy.
2. Pour into glasses and serve foamy, or strain through a strainer to remove the pulp before serving over ice.

Notes: Add one shot of vodka, tequila, or rum per serving for a spicier version.

Nutrition Facts: Calories: 129 | Carbohydrates: 33 g | Protein: 1 g | Fat: 9 g | Cholesterol: 100 mg

164. SOUTHERN ORANGEADE RECIPE

Prep Time: 10 minutes
Cook Time: 3 minutes
Total Time: 13 minutes
Servings: 8

Ingredients:
- Two 1/2 cups of fresh-squeezed orange juice from 6-8 juicy oranges
- 1/2 cups granulated sugar
- 1/2 cups water
- 1/2 cup fresh squeezed lemon juice
- 1/4 teaspoon vanilla extract
- Pinch of salt
- 5 cups club soda or water

Directions:
1. In a small sauce saucepan, combine 1 1/2 cups sugar and 1 1/2 cups water. Heat and stir until all of the sugar has dissolved. (You can also do this in the microwave.) Add the vanilla extract and a sprinkle of salt and mix well.
2. In a large pitcher, combine 2 1/2 cups orange juice and 1/2 cup lemon juice. Fill the pitcher halfway with sugar syrup. If you're making it ahead of time, add 5 cups of water. Refrigerate after stirring.
3. Pour 5 cups of club soda into the pitcher instead of tap water if serving right immediately. This produces a frothy soda fountain effect!

Notes: Orangeade tastes best when made with ripe, juicy oranges. I like to use a combination of Cara Cara and Navel oranges.

Nutrition Facts: Calories: 183 | Carbohydrates: 46 g | Protein: 0 g | Fat: 0 g | Cholesterol: 44 mg

165. VODKA GUMMY BEARS POPSICLES

Prep Time: 20 minutes
Cook Time: 320 minutes
Total Time: 340 minutes
Servings: 10

Ingredients:
- 1/4 cup vodka
- 1/4 cup gummy bears
- 2 cups Sprite ginger ale or Fanta! work well too
- Wooden popsicle sticks

Directions:
1. Pour the vodka into a mixing bowl. Add the gummy bears, cover, and soak for 24 to 72 hours. The more alcohol the gummy bears absorb, the longer they soak. They are also growing in size!
2. Stir to separate the gummy bears after they have soaked to your preference. Then separate one-third of them from the vodka and pour into the bottoms of ten popsicle molds. Pour Sprite over the gummy bears until they are barely coated, approximately a third of the way full. After that, place in the freezer for 60-90 minutes.
3. After the initial layer has frozen, add the popsicle sticks, followed by a second layer of strained gummy bears and soda. Freeze once more, then repeat three times. The entire layering/freezing time should be 4+ hours.

Notes: Omit the alcohol and soaking procedure for a kid-friendly version.

Nutrition Facts: Calories: 102 | Carbohydrates: 8 g | Protein: 1 g | Fat: 0 g | Cholesterol: 26 mg

166. BAILEYS IRISH CREAM JELLO SHOTS

Prep Time: 5 minutes
Cook Time: 3 minutes
Total Time: 8 minutes
Servings: 8

Ingredients:
- 750 ml Bailey's Irish Cream liqueur (1 bottle)
- 2 cups hot coffee or espresso
- 5 packets unflavored gelatin, divided

- 3 tablespoons granulated sugar
- whipped cream

Directions:
1. Wrap a 9X9 baking dish in plastic wrap. Fill a medium dish halfway with hot coffee. Stir in the sugar. Then mix in 2 packets of unflavored gelatin quickly. Make sure there are no clumps by whisking quickly. Pour the coffee gelatin into the pan that has been prepared. Refrigerate for at least 1 hour or until the mixture is stiff. Then, using a wooden stick, poke holes in the gelatin's surface. (This will aid in the adhesion of the two gelatin layers.)
2. 1 cup Baileys Irish Cream, heated on the stovetop or in a microwave-safe dish Heat until almost boiling, then mix in 3 packets unflavored gelatin, ensuring no clumps. Then, whisk in the remainder of the bottle of Baileys. Pour the Baileys gelatin over the coffee gelatin and mix well. Refrigerate for at least 2 hours, or until the mixture is fully solid.
3. Lift the entire sheet of gelatin out of the pan using the plastic wrap's edges. Make 36 squares out of the gelatin. To produce round jello shots, use a tiny 1 - 1 ½ inch cooker cutter.
4. Top each jello shot with a tiny dollop of whipped cream. Put it in the fridge until you're ready to serve it.

Nutrition Facts: Calories: 83 | Carbohydrates: 10 g | Protein: 0 g | Fat: 0 g | Cholesterol: 0 mg

167. **AFFOGATO BOURBON SHOTS**

Prep Time: 2 minutes
Cook Time: 2 minutes
Total Time: 4 minutes
Servings: 1

Ingredients:
- 1/2 tablespoon vanilla gelato or ice cream
- 3/4 ounce bourbon
- 3/4 ounce chilled espresso

Directions:
1. Make enough espresso to make as many Affogato Bourbon Shots as you like. The espresso should then be chilled.
2. Fill 2-ounce shot glasses halfway with tiny ice cream balls.
3. Pour the cooled espresso over the ice cream, then the bourbon. Serve right away.

Nutrition Facts: Calories: 96 | Carbohydrates: 5 g | Protein: 0 g | Fat: 1 g | Cholesterol: 19 mg

168. **HIBISCUS GINGER ICED TEA AND MARTINI**

Prep Time: 5 minutes
Cook Time: 5 minutes
Total Time: 10 minutes
Servings: 4

Ingredients:
Hibiscus Ginger Iced Tea
- Four quarts of water
- 3-4 slices of fresh ginger, (no need to peel)
- 3/4 cup of dried hibiscus flowers (about 1 large handful)
- 3/4 to 1 cup sugar

Hibiscus-Ginger Simple Syrup
- Two inch ginger piece (Cut thinly)
- 1/2 cups water
- 1/2 cups sugar
- 3/4 cup dried hibiscus flowers
- Hibiscus Ginger Martini
- ounce Hibiscus-Ginger Simple Syrup
- ounce vodka or gin
- 2+ oz seltzer or club soda
- Garnish: pieces of ginger and rehydrated flowers

Directions:
Hibiscus Ginger Iced Tea
1. In a big pot, add water, ginger, and dried hibiscus blossoms.
2. Bring a pot of water to a boil. Allow the ginger and hibiscus flowers to boiling for 3-5 minutes in the water.

3. Allow the tea to cool to room temperature. The ginger and dried flowers are then strained out.
4. Serve with ice.

Hibiscus-Ginger Simple Syrup
1. Thinly slice a 2 inch piece of ginger. (There is no need to peel)
2. In a small saucepan, combine 1 ½ cups water, 1 ½ cups sugar, 1 big handful of dried hibiscus flowers, and the sliced ginger.
3. Bring the water to a boil. Remove from the heat and cover.
4. Allow to steep until the infusion has cooled to room temperature. Reserving some of the flowers and ginger for garnishes, strain out the flowers and ginger.

Hibiscus Ginger Martini
1. Shaken — combine the hibiscus-ginger simple syrup, vodka/gin, and club soda/seltzer in a cocktail shaker. Shake a few times before straining into a martini glass.
2. Stirred – Combine the hibiscus-ginger simple syrup, vodka/gin, and club soda/seltzer in a small glass. Stir everything together until well combined, then strain into a martini glass.
3. Garnish on top for a little more flare!

Notes:
There are many ways to use that hibiscus ginger simple syrup; have fun with it and let me know what wonderful dishes you come up with!

Nutrition Facts: Calories: 162 | Carbohydrates: 41 g | Protein: 24 g | Fat: 18 g | Cholesterol: 98 mg

169. **CHOCOLATE BRANDY LATTE**

Prep Time: 2 minutes
Cook Time: 3 minutes
Total Time: 5 minutes
Servings: 2

Ingredients:
- 2 oz hot espresso
- 2 oz Kohler Dark Chocolate Brandy
- ¾ cup steamed whole milk, or half & half
- 1 tablespoon turbinado sugar
- Optional garnishes: whipped cream and chocolate syrup

Directions:
1. Fill a tall tumbler halfway with hot espresso. Stir in the sugar to dissolve it.
2. Pour in the heated milk and Kohler Dark Chocolate Brandy. Stir.
3. If desired, garnish with whipped cream and chocolate syrup.

Notes: You can prepare steamed milk in the microwave if you don't have a milk steamer. Fill a mason jar halfway with milk. Screw on the lid and violently shake for 30 seconds. Remove the cover and microwave for 30 seconds to let the foam solidify.

Nutrition Facts: Calories: 147 | Carbohydrates: 10 g | Protein: 3 g | Fat: 5 g | Cholesterol: 9 mg

170. **TOFFEE CARAMEL LATTE**

Prep Time: 3 minutes
Cook Time: 3 minutes
Total Time: 6 minutes
Servings: 1

Ingredients:
- 4 tablespoons of espresso 2 shots
- ¾ cup of steamed milk
- ½ tablespoons of toffee nut syrup
- ¾ tablespoon of caramel sauce
- Whipped cream and caramel sauce to garnish

Directions:
1. Pour heated milk and espresso into a 10-ounce cup.
2. Combine the toffee syrup and caramel sauce in a mixing bowl.
3. Whipped cream and additional caramel sauce on top.

Nutrition Facts: Calories: 231 | Carbohydrates: 39 g | Protein: 24 g | Fat: 6 g | Cholesterol: 37 mg

CHAPTER 8: SNACKS (CLEAR FLUIDS)

171. LEMON RICOTTA CAKE (CREPE CAKE RECIPE)

Prep Time: 20 minutes
Cook Time: 25 minutes
Total Time: 45 minutes
Servings: 16

Ingredients:
For the Ricotta Cream Filling
- 1/4 cups heavy cream
- 1/2 cup granulated sugar
- teaspoon vanilla extract
- 32 oz ricotta cheese

For the Strawberry Sauce
- 3 cups fresh strawberries, hulled and divided
- 1/3 cup strawberry jam
- Pinch salt
- Chopped pistachios, optional garnish

For the Crepe Batter
- tablespoons melted butter
- 2/3 cups whole milk
- 1/4 cups water
- 2 1/2 cups all-purpose flour
- 3 tablespoons granulated sugar
- 1/2 teaspoons salt
- 5 large eggs
- Zest of 1 lemon + 1 tablespoon juice

Directions:
For the Ricotta Cream Filling
1. In a mixing bowl, combine the ricotta cheese. Fill a Vita-mix Blender container halfway with heavy cream, sugar, and vanilla extract. Cover and push the "Start" button at level 1. Increase the speed of the machine to level 10 by turning it on. For gentle peaks, blend for 10-15 seconds. Don't over mix, or you'll end up with churned butter!
2. Scoop the whipped cream from the blender jar and mix it gently into the ricotta cheese with a spatula. (If you put the ricotta in the blender, it will crumble.) Place in the refrigerator until ready to use.

For the Strawberry Sauce
1. Rinse the blender jar well. To the jar, add 2 cups cut strawberries, strawberry jam, and a sprinkle of salt: blend and cover. Begin with level 1 and gradually increase the speed until the strawberries are dissolved. Refrigerate the strawberry sauce in a small jar until ready to serve.

For the Crepe Batter
1. Rinse the blender jar well. Combine the flour, sugar, salt, eggs, milk, water, melted butter, 1 lemon zest, and 1 tablespoon lemon juice in a mixing bowl. Cover and mix for 5 seconds on level 1. Then, gradually raise the speed to level 10, until the mixture is foamy. If there are visible flour clumps, scrape the jar's edges. Then, cover and mix for another 5-10 seconds.
2. Over medium heat, heat a 9- to 10-inch flat nonstick crepe pan. Once the pan is heated, spoon batter into the center of the crepe pan with a 1/4-cup scoop. Lift and swirl the pan quickly to form a thin 9-inch circle of batter. Return the pan to the stovetop. If you're having problems forming uniform circles, use a spatula to transfer the batter to the pan's sparse spots swiftly.
3. Cook for 30-40 seconds on each side, turning with a broad flat spatula. The first side should have a light golden hue with golden speckles, and the second side should be lighter. Turn the heat up to medium-high if your crepes are taking longer than 90 seconds total per crepe.

4. Repeat with the remaining crepes on a baking sheet (or plate) coated with parchment paper. The crepes will be brittle at first, but they will soften in a matter of minutes. You should have 20-24 crepes. It is OK to stack them on the sheet. They will not cling together if they are thoroughly cooked.
5. Before proceeding, allow the crepes to cool fully. To expedite the chilling process, place the baking sheet in the refrigerator.

To Assemble
1. Begin building the cake after the crepes have completely cooled. One crepe should be placed on a cake stand. Spread 1/4 cup ricotta filling in a thin circle over the crepe, leaving a 1/2-inch ring around the edges without cream. Repeat with the remaining crepes. Spread ricotta cream and stack crepes until all of the ricotta filling and/or crepes are used. To level out the layers, use a flat plate or baking sheet to push down on the top of the cake. Cover loosely with plastic wrap and keep refrigerated until ready to serve.

To Serve
1. Slice the remaining 1 cup fresh strawberries and put them on top of the cake. Pour some of the strawberry sauce over the strawberries, allowing it to drip down the edges. The leftover sauce should be reserved for pouring over individual slices of cake. If desired, decorate the top of the cake with chopped pistachios.
2. When it's time to cut the cake, use a serrated knife and make nice, even slices with a gently sawing motion. Serve with more strawberry sauce.

Nutrition Facts: Calories: 349 | Carbohydrates: 53 g | Protein: 48 g | Fat: 2 g | Cholesterol: 284 mg

Servings: 6

Ingredients:
- 3 very ripe plantains yellow with lots of blacks
- 6 tablespoons butter
- clove garlic smashed
- Salt

Directions:
1. Remove the plantain tips. Peel the plantains and cut them into 12 inch thick ovals at an angle.
2. Preheat a big sauté pan or cast iron skillet to medium heat. Then, on the side, place a "holding plate" lined with paper towels.
3. Melt the butter in the pan. Once the butter has melted, add the crushed garlic clove and plantain pieces in a single layer to the pan. (Depending on the size of your pan, you may need to do this in two batches.) Fry the plantains until golden brown, about 2-3 minutes per side.
4. When the plantains are golden and crisp, transfer them to a holding plate with a slotted spoon. Season generously with salt. If necessary, repeat with the remaining plantains.
5. Remove the garlic clove. Warm it up with your favorite Mexican or Caribbean dishes!

Notes: Be careful to use plenty of ripe plantains... They should be dark or have big black dots if they are fully ripe. When eaten immediately after being fried, fried plantains offer the finest texture and flavor. However, when they've cooled, you may store leftover plantains in an airtight jar in the fridge for up to 3 days. Reheat in the oven, toaster, or on the stovetop. I do not advocate freezing fried sweet plantains.

Nutrition Facts: Calories: 210 | Carbohydrates: 29 g | Protein: 17 g | Fat: 22 g | Cholesterol: 187 mg

172. **SWEET FRIED PLANTAINS**

Prep Time: 5 minutes
Cook Time: 5 minutes
Total Time: 10 minutes

173. **MANGO PUDDING (DAIRY FREE!) RECIPE**

Prep Time: 15 minutes

Cook Time: 5 minutes
Total Time: 20 minutes
Servings: 11

Ingredients:
- Two cups of mango puree from 2 large juicy mangos
- 13.5 ounce can unsweetened coconut milk
- One cup of hot water
- One cup of granulated sugar
- Five teaspoons of unflavored gelatin powder measured from 2 packets
- One teaspoon of vanilla extract
- One pinches salt

Directions:
1. Place a big liquid measuring cup on the table. Combine the boiling water, sugar, gelatin, and salt in a mixing bowl. Allow the mixture to rest for 5 minutes after thoroughly stirring.
2. Meanwhile, peel and chop the mangoes into big bits. Remove the pits and peels. In a blender, combine the mango pieces. Puree till smooth, then measure out 2 cups. (If necessary, scoop some out of the mixer.)
3. Blend in the coconut milk and vanilla extract. Blend until smooth. Then add the gelatin mixture to the blender and blend until smooth. Puree one more until smooth.
4. Fill tiny 4 ounce serving glasses halfway with mango pudding. To set, cover and refrigerate the cups for 3-4 hours. Garnish with mint and serve chilled. Garnish with toasted coconut, lime zest, or chopped cashews if desired.

Note: You may alternatively use frozen mango pieces that have been thawed. Store in the refrigerator, covered, for up to 5 days.

Nutrition Facts: Calories: 174 | Carbohydrates: 26 g | Protein: 18 g | Fat: 8 g | Cholesterol: 281 mg

174. FRENCH CHOCOLATE SILK PIE RECIPE

Prep Time: 30 minutes
Cook Time: 15 minutes
Total Time: 45 minutes
Servings: 10

Ingredients:
- unbaked pie crust, store-bought or homemade
- 6 oz bittersweet chocolate + extra for shavings
- 1/2 cups of heavy cream
- One cup of unsalted butter softened (2 sticks)
- One cup of granulated sugar, divided
- ½ teaspoons of vanilla extract
- 1/2 teaspoon of salt
- large pasteurized eggs

Directions:
1. Preheat the oven to 375 degrees Fahrenheit. Fill a large 9-inch pie pan halfway with pie dough. The edges should be crimped. Then, cover the pie shell with parchment paper and fill it with dry beans or ceramic pie weights. Cook for 15-20 minutes, or until the edges are golden brown. Allow the pie crust to cool fully after removing the parchment containing the weights.
2. Meanwhile, in a double boiler, melt 6 oz of chocolate. When the chocolate has melted, remove it from the heat and let it cool to room temperature.
3. In the bowl of an electric mixer, combine the heavy cream and 1/4 cup sugar. Whip the cream on high with a whip attachment until it forms firm peaks. Place the whipped cream in a separate dish and set aside until ready to use.

4. Using the same mixer bowl and a paddle attachment, beat the butter and 3/4 cup sugar on high for at least 3 minutes, or until light and fluffy. Turn the heat to low and gradually add the cooled chocolate to the butter mixture, vanilla, and salt. Scrape down the mixer bowl and continue to beat until smooth.
5. Increase the speed of the mixer to high. Add 1 egg at a time, allowing the mixer to beat the egg for at least 3 minutes before adding the next egg. This results in a super-smooth texture. After 12 minutes on high, switch off the mixer. Using a spatula, gently fold in 1/3 of the whipped cream. Fold until the mixture is smooth.
6. Fill the cooled pie shell with the chocolate mixture. Serve with the remaining whipped cream on top. Then, using a vegetable peeler, shave chocolate over the top. Refrigerate for at least 3 hours, or until the chocolate filling has firmed up.

Nutrition Facts: Calories: 549 | Carbohydrates: 30 g | Protein: 54 g | Fat: 28 g | Cholesterol: 197 mg

175. **PEANUT BUTTER OATMEAL CHOCOLATE CHIP COOKIES (MONSTER COOKIE RECIPE)**

Prep Time: 15 minutes
Cook Time: 15 minutes
Total Time: 30 minutes
Servings: 55

Ingredients:
- 5 ½ cups rolled oats (gluten free)
- 5 large eggs
- ¼ cup water
- 2 tablespoons of vanilla extract
- One cup of unsalted butter, softened (2 sticks)
- ¾ cups peanut butter, crunchy or creamy
- ½ cups granulated sugar
- ½ cups light brown sugar, packed
- ½ cup all-purpose flour (or GF baking flour)
- 4 tablespoon baking powder
- 1 teaspoon salt
- 12 ounce semi-sweet chocolate chips
- 12 ounce M&Ms

Directions:
1. Preheat the oven to 350 degrees Fahrenheit. Set aside several baking sheets lined with parchment paper.
2. Measure out the oats in a large mixing basin. Then, crack the eggs into the oats and stir in the water and vanilla extract. Allow the liquid to soak the oats before stirring to coat.
3. Add the butter to the bowl of an electric stand mixer. To soften, beat for 1 minute. After that, stir in the peanut butter and both sugars. To break down the sugar crystals, beat on high for 3-5 minutes.
4. Scrape down the sides of the bowl with a spatula and beat again to incorporate.
5. Mix in the flour, baking powder, and salt with the mixer on low. Begin adding the oat mixture once everything has been thoroughly combined.
6. Scrape the bowl one more, then mix in the chocolate chips on low.
7. Finally, using a spatula, fold the M&Ms into the dough.
8. To distribute the cookie dough onto the prepared baking sheets, use a big 3 tablespoon cookie scoop. Place the cookies 2 inches apart on a baking sheet.
9. Bake for 15-17 minutes each batch, or until the edges are just starting to turn golden brown. Cool for 3 minutes on the baking sheets before transferring.

Nutrition Facts: Calories: 230 | Carbohydrates: 26 g | Protein: 4 g | Fat: 7 g | Cholesterol: 18 mg

176. BANANA OATMEAL CHOCOLATE CHIP COOKIES (HEALTHY!)

Prep Time: 15 minutes
Cook Time: 12 minutes
Total Time: 27 minutes
Servings: 18

Ingredients:
- Two cups quick oats
- ½ cups almond flour
- 3 large brown bananas mashed (about 1 cup)
- ½ cup light brown sugar or palm sugar
- large egg
- Two teaspoons of baking powder
- One teaspoon vanilla extract
- ¼ teaspoon salt
- ¼ cups dark chocolate chips

Directions:
1. Preheat the oven to 350 degrees Fahrenheit. 2 big baking sheets, lined with parchment paper
2. Combine the oats, almond flour, mashed bananas, brown sugar, egg, baking powder, vanilla extract, and salt in an electric stand mixer bowl. Beat the mixture until it is smooth and uniform.
3. Then, with the mixer on low, fold in HALF of the chocolate chips.
4. To distribute the cookies onto the baking pans, use a 1.5 tablespoon cookie scoop. Set them apart by 2 inches.
5. Place 4-5 chocolate chips on top of each cookie, flattening the dough balls slightly.
6. Bake for 12 minutes or until the edges are firm. Cool for 5 minutes on the cookie sheets before transferring.

Nutrition Facts: Calories: 192 | Carbohydrates: 24 g | Protein: 51 g | Fat: 9 g | Cholesterol: 261 mg

177. LARABAR SNACK BAR

Prep Time: 5 minutes
Cook Time: 5 minutes
Total Time: 10 minutes
Servings: 12

Ingredients:
- 2 cup raw almonds
- 3/4 cup pitted dates packed
- 1 cup dried unsweetened apples
- 1/4 cup raisins packed
- 1/2 teaspoon cinnamon
- 1/4 teaspoon sea salt

Directions:
1. In a food processor, combine all of the ingredients and process until finely chopped and sticky.
2. Line an 8-inch baking dish with wax paper, leaving enough to hang over the sides to cover the mixture. Fill the dish halfway with the mixture and top with wax paper. Press or roll out the ingredients until it is smooth.
3. Remove the wax paper and bars from the pan and cut them into 12 equal bars. Wrap each piece in wax paper and store it in an airtight container.

Nutrition Facts: Calories: 153 | Carbohydrates: 17 g | Protein: 17 g | Fat: 27 g | Cholesterol: 89 mg

178. KULFI INDIAN ICE CREAM

Prep Time: 10 minutes
Cook Time: 160 minutes
Total Time: 170 minutes
Servings: 16

Ingredients:
- 2 cups heavy cream
- 14 ounces can sweeten condensed milk
- 2 teaspoon ground cardamom
- 1 teaspoon vanilla extract
- ½ cup chopped pistachios
- 1 pinch saffron + 1 tbs warm water

Directions:

1. In a small dish, combine 1 tablespoon hot tap water. Allow a pinch of saffron to soak to absorb its color and taste.
2. Meanwhile, prepare an electric mixer fitted with a whip attachment. Pour in the heavy cream, cardamom powder, and vanilla essence. Whip the mixture at high speed until firm peaks form.
3. Using a rubber spatula, scrape the bowl. Then add the saffron and water and mix well.
4. Fold in the sweetened condensed milk using a spatula. Fold in the chopped pistachios after the mixture is smooth and uniform.
5. Insert the kulfi in an airtight container and freeze it, or spoon it into tiny cups for popsicles and place a popsicle stick in the center of each one.
6. Freeze for a minimum of 3 hours.

Nutrition Facts: Calories: 200 | Carbohydrates: 16 g | Protein: 14 g | Fat: 18 g | Cholesterol: 44 mg

179. **EASY NO-BAKE KEY LIME PIE RECIPE**

Prep Time: 20 minutes
Cook Time: 240 minutes
Total Time: 260 minutes
Servings: 8

Ingredients:
For the Graham Cracker Crust
- 12 whole graham crackers crushed (about 1 ½ cups)
- Six tablespoons melted butter
- ¼ cup granulated sugar
- ¼ teaspoon salt

For the Key Lime Pie Filling
- Eight ounce cream cheese softened
- 14 ounce sweetened condensed milk
- ½ cup key lime juice
- 3-5 drops lime green food coloring if desired
- 8 ounce Cool Whip
- Lime zest for garnish

Directions:
1. Prepare a 9-inch pie pan as well as a food processor. In a food processor, combine the graham crackers. Close the lid and pulse into a fine crumb. After that, stir in the melted butter, sugar, and salt. To mix, pulse the ingredients together.
2. Fill the pie pan halfway with the graham cracker crumble. Press it into an equal layer over the bottom and up the edges of the pan with your hands. Keep refrigerated until ready to use.
3. Wipe the food processor bowl clean. Then combine the cream cheese, sweetened condensed milk, and lime juice in a mixing bowl. Blend until smooth. (If wanted, add food coloring here.)
4. Take the food processor blade out of the machine. Scoop the Cool Whip into the lime mixture and stir well. Fold the Cool Whip into the mixture with a spatula until completely smooth.
5. Fill the pie crust with the filling. Then, store the mixture in the freezer for at least 4 hours, undisturbed.
6. If preferred, top with fresh lime zest when ready to serve. While still frozen, cut into pieces. Allow each piece to remain at room temperature for 10 minutes before serving somewhat softened.

Nutrition Facts: Calories: 451 | Carbohydrates: 60 g | Protein: 63 g | Fat: 28 g | Cholesterol: 59 mg

180. **LEMON CHEESECAKE RECIPE (LIMONCELLO CAKE!)**

Prep Time: 20 minutes
Cook Time: 60 minutes
Total Time: 80 minutes
Servings: 16

Ingredients:
For the Biscoff Crust
- 8.8 oz Biscoff Cookies, 1 package
- 1/2 cup granulated sugar

- 1/2 teaspoon salt
- 1/2 cup unsalted butter, melted

For the Limoncello Cheesecake Filling
- 24 oz cream cheese, softened
- 4 large eggs
- 3/4 cup granulated sugar
- 1 large lemon, zested and juiced (1/4 cup juice)
- 1/4 cup limoncello liqueur
- 1/2 teaspoon vanilla extract
- 1/2 teaspoon salt

For the Sour Cream Topping
- 16 oz sour cream
- 1/4 cup granulated sugar
- 3 tablespoons limoncello liqueur

Directions:
1. Preheat the oven to 350 degrees Fahrenheit. Place one oven rack in the center and one at the bottom of the oven. To catch any spillage, use a big rimmed baking sheet on the bottom rack. Preheat the oven to 350°F. Line the bottom of a 9 1/2-inch springform pan with parchment paper. Then, securely tighten the ring around the bottom. (If desired, trim the paper edges.)
2. To make the Crust: In a food processor, combine the Biscoff cookies, sugar, and salt. Pulse the cookies until they are finely ground. After that, add the melted butter and pulse to the mix. Fill the prepared pan halfway with the crust mixture. With your hands, press the crumbs all over the bottom of the pan and approximately two-thirds of the way up the edges. 10 minutes in the oven
3. Meanwhile, prepare the Limoncello Cheesecake Filling by placing the cream cheese in the bowl of an electric mixer. 2 minutes on high to soften and fluff the cream cheese. Add the eggs one at a time, delaying adding another until the preceding egg is thoroughly mixed in. Using a spatula, scrape the bowl. Then mix in the other ingredients until fully smooth—Bake for 45 minutes after pouring the filling into the crust.
4. To make the Sour Cream Topping, combine the sour cream, sugar, and limoncello in a medium mixing bowl and whisk until smooth. Once the cheesecake has baked and is nearly set in the center, pour the sour cream filling over the top and return to the oven for 10-12 minutes.
5. 1 hour on the counter to cool the cheesecake. Then place in the refrigerator for at least 3 hours to cool. Remove the ring from the springform pan and place the cheesecake on a cake plate. Cut into slices and serve chilled.

Nutrition Facts: Calories: 386 | Carbohydrates: 35 g | Protein: 22 g | Fat: 17 g | Cholesterol: 108 mg

181. **FRENCH TOAST**

Prep Time: 10 minutes
Cook Time: 25 minutes
Total Time: 35 minutes
Servings: 10

Ingredients:
- One loaf brioche bread, unsliced
- Two cups half & half
- Five egg yolks
- 1/2 cups granulated sugar
- 1 teaspoon vanilla extract
- One pinches salt
- Six tablespoons butter
- Possible Toppings: Toasted almonds, fresh berries, powdered sugar, maple syrup, caramel sauce, chocolate shavings

Directions:
1. Preheat the oven to 275°F. Prepare a big baking sheet.
2. Combine the half-and-half, egg yolks, sugar, vanilla, and salt in a large mixing bowl. Make sure the sugar is completely dissolved.
3. Slice the brioche bread into 1 inch pieces using a serrated knife. (Approximately 10 slices.)

4. Preheat a large skillet over medium-high heat. Depending on the size of the skillet, add 1-2 tablespoons of butter.
5. Soak 2-3 brioche slices in the egg mixture for 30-60 seconds, turning to coat. The bread should soak for just long enough to be completely soaked, but not so long that it dissolves.
6. Transfer the wet bread to the heated skillet with care. Fry the pieces of French toast for 2-3 minutes per side, or until golden brown. If they're cooking too quickly, reduce the heat to medium-low to ensure the interior is cooked through the middle.
7. Place the French toast on a baking pan and keep warm in the oven. (The longer it bakes, the puffier it will get.)
8. Wipe out the skillet with a paper towel and add additional butter to it. (Wipe the skillet only if the butter residue becomes black.)
9. Repeat with the remaining bread pieces until all of the French Toast is made. Put one batch in the oven at a time to keep it warm.
10. Serve warm with fresh berries, maple syrup, or other toppings of your choice!

Nutrition Facts: Calories: 369 | Carbohydrates: 29 g | Protein: 8 g | Fat: 25 g | Cholesterol: 210 mg

182. **PINEAPPLE ORANGE CREAMSICLE**

Prep Time: 10 minutes
Cook Time: 12 minutes
Total Time: 22 minutes
Servings: 10

Ingredients:
- Two cups of orange-pineapple juice
- One cup heavy cream
- ½ cup granulated sugar
- 2 teaspoons vanilla extract

Directions:

1. In a microwave-safe bowl, combine 1/2 cup juice and 1/2 sugar. Warm the juice for 1-2 minutes or until the sugar melts. Then add the remaining juice and whisk to combine.
2. Pour the heavy cream, vanilla extract, and 1 1/4 cup of the sweetened juice into a separate dish (or measuring pitcher). Stir everything together thoroughly. Then divide the mixture evenly among ten regular popsicle molds.
3. For 1 hour, place the popsicles in the freezer. Then, drizzle the remaining juice over the tops of each popsicle and insert wooden popsicle sticks. Freeze for at least 3 hours more.

Nutrition Facts: Calories: 145 | Carbohydrates: 15 g | Protein: 17 g | Fat: 8 g | Cholesterol: 76 mg

183. **EASY PEACH COBBLER RECIPE WITH BISQUICK**

Prep Time: 10 minutes
Cook Time: 60 minutes
Total Time: 70 minutes
Servings: 7

Ingredients:
- 48 oz fresh or frozen sliced peaches 6 ½ cups, with or without peels
- Two cups granulated sugar
- ½ teaspoon of pumpkin pie spice or apple pie spice blend
- cups Bisquick baking mix
- 1 cup of whole milk
- 1 cup of melted butter

Directions:

1. Preheat the oven to 350 degrees Fahrenheit. Prepare a 9-by-13-inch baking dish and a large mixing basin.

2. If you are using fresh peaches, cut them into wedges and remove the pits. Fill the baking dish halfway with fresh (or frozen) peach slices. Then, over the peaches, add 1 cup sugar and the pumpkin pie spice. Toss the peach to coat it, then spread it out in an equal layer.
3. Combine the remaining 1 cup sugar, Bisquick, and milk in a mixing basin. Whisk everything together well. Then add the melted butter and stir until combined.
4. Pour the batter over the peaches in an equal layer. Bake for 55- 60 minutes, depending on the size of the baking dish.
5. After 40 minutes, check on the cobbler. If the top begins to darken, loosely cover with foil and continue baking.
6. Allow at least 15 minutes for the cobbler to cool before serving. Serve in dishes with vanilla ice cream or whipped cream.

Notes: You don't like peaches? Replace the nectarines, plums, pitted cherries, or berries with an equal number of nectarines, plums, pitted cherries, or berries in this recipe.

How to Keep Leftovers: Once the cobbler has completely cooled, cover it in plastic wrap or move it to a container with a lid. The fruit cobbler may be stored in the refrigerator for up to 4-5 days.

To put on ice: Cook according to the recipe in a freezer-safe baking dish, cool, and cover the entire dish in plastic wrap. Wrap in tin foil and place in the freezer for up to 3 months. Unwrap and bake in a 350°F oven for 40-50 minutes, or until boiling.

Nutrition Facts: Calories: 420 | Carbohydrates: 59 g | Protein: 11 g | Fat: 20 g | Cholesterol: 172 mg

184. **HEALTHY 5-MINUTE STRAWBERRY PINEAPPLE SHERBET**

Prep Time: 5 minutes
Cook Time: 5 minutes
Total Time: 10 minutes
Servings: 16

Ingredients:
- One pound frozen strawberries
- One pound has frozen pineapple chunks
- 1/2 cups plain Greek yogurt
- 1/2 cup honey or palm syrup
- Two teaspoon vanilla extract
- Pinch salt

Directions:
1. In a large food mixer, combine all of the ingredients. Pulse the frozen fruit to break it up. Then purée until completely smooth.
2. Serve immediately as soft serve, or freeze in an airtight container. Thaw for 15 minutes before scooping and serving if frozen.

Notes: This sherbet has a distinct honey taste. If you dislike the flavor of honey, use palm syrup.

Nutrition Facts: Calories: 70 | Carbohydrates: 16 g | Protein: 2 g | Fat: 1 g | Cholesterol: 1 mg

185. **BEST COCONUT MILK ICE CREAM (DAIRY-FREE!)**

Prep Time: 3 minutes
Cook Time: 30 minutes
Total Time: 33 minutes
Servings: 16

Ingredients:
- 27 ounce canned full-fat unsweetened coconut milk 2 cans
- 13.6 ounce can coconut cream
- One cup granulated sugar
- Two teaspoons of vanilla extract or vanilla bean paste
- ¼ teaspoon salt

Directions:

1. After making this ice cream numerous times, I learned that it does not always need to be heated/cooked before churning... This saves a huge amount of time. (This depends on the kind of coconut milk/cream and the kind of blender you use.) Put all ingredients in a blender and purée until smooth to see whether your ice cream has to be cooked. If the coconut ice cream mixture is smooth and free of clumps, you may churn it without heating.
2. Heat and stir: If there are any pieces of coconut cream in the recipe, they will freeze as hard waxy clumps in the ice cream. In this scenario, cook the mixture over medium heat until smooth, stirring often. Before churning, chill and cool to at least room temperature. * If you don't want to "test" the no-heat approach, simply combine all ingredients in a saucepot and cook over medium heat until smooth, allowing the coconut clumps and sugar to dissolve. Then take a break.
3. Set out a 1.5-2 quart ice cream machine after the ice cream mixture has cooled. Turn on the machine and place the frozen bowl inside. Fill the machine halfway with the extremely smooth ice cream mixture. Cook for 20-25 minutes, or until the mixture is thick, hard, and smooth.
4. Serve right away, or transfer to an airtight container and freeze until ready to use.

Nutrition Facts: Calories: 224 | Carbohydrates: 16 g | Protein: 2 g | Fat: 19 g | Cholesterol: 27 mg

186. **LEMON CRINKLE COOKIES RECIPE**

Prep Time: 15 minutes
Cook Time: 10 minutes
Total Time: 25 minutes
Servings: 45

Ingredients:

- 1 cup unsalted butter, softened (2 sticks)
- ¾ cups granulated sugar
- 4 large eggs
- 2 tablespoons fresh lemon juice
- 2 tablespoon lemon zest
- 1 teaspoon vanilla extract
- 1 cup all-purpose flour (stir, spoon into the cup, and level)
- 2 teaspoon baking powder
- 1/2 teaspoon salt
- 1/4 teaspoon baking soda
- 2-5 drops yellow food coloring (optional)
- 2 cup powdered sugar

Directions:
1. In the bowl of an electric stand mixer, combine the butter and granulated sugar. Cream the butter and sugar together on high for 3-5 minutes, or until light and creamy. Using a rubber spatula, scrape the bowl.
2. Mix in the eggs, lemon juice, lemon zest, and vanilla extract at low speed. Scrape the bowl once more. Mix in 1 cup of flour, baking powder, salt, baking soda, and food coloring on low. Once mixed, gently fold in the remaining 2 cups of flour until smooth. (Be careful not to overwork the dough!)
3. Refrigerate the dough for at least 30 minutes, covered. (The longer the dough is chilled, the puffier the cookies.) Preheat the oven to 375 degrees Fahrenheit. Set aside several baking sheets lined with parchment paper.
4. Set out a small dish of powdered sugar once the dough has cooled. To separate the dough into balls, use a 1 tablespoon cookie scoop. Roll each ball in powdered sugar, then place 2 inches apart on baking pans. (Be careful to cover the cookies with powdered sugar generously.) You should not shrug them off.)
5. 9-10 minutes, or until the sides are golden brown and the middle appears slightly underbaked. Allow them to cool on the baking pans so that the centers continue to bake as they cool.

Note: Storage Suggestions: Store the cookies in an airtight jar at room temperature. Consume within 7-10 days.
Citrus Substitutions: In place of the lemon, you can use lime or orange juice and zest. You may also combine lemon and lime for a unique taste combination!
Nutrition Facts: Calories: 111 | Carbohydrates: 16 g | Protein: 29 g | Fat: 18 g | Cholesterol: 63 mg

187. THE BEST NO-BAKE CHOCOLATE LASAGNA

Prep Time: 20 minutes
Cook Time: 120 minutes
Total Time: 140 minutes
Servings: 12

Ingredients:
Oreo Layer
- 40 Oreo cookies
- 7 tablespoons melted butter
- Cream Cheese Layer –
- 8 oz cream cheese softened
- 3 tablespoons granulated sugar
- Two tablespoons of milk
- 16 oz of Cool whip reserve half for later

Chocolate Pudding Layer
- 7.8 oz instant chocolate pudding mix two small boxes
- 2 ¾ cups of milk
- Two teaspoons instant coffee granules
- Whipped Topping Layer –
- Remaining Cool Whip
- 2 cup mini chocolate chips or ½ cup chocolate shavings

Directions:
1. Set up a big food processor to make the Oreo crust. In a mixing dish, combine the Oreo cookies. Cover and pulse until tiny crumbs form. Then, pulse in the melted butter to coat. * If you don't have a food processor, you may smash the cookies with a rolling pin in a zip bag. Then, for the remaining processes, use a mixer.
2. Fill a 9 x 13 inch baking dish halfway with Oreo crumbs. Chill after pressing into a uniform layer.
3. A layer of Cream Cheese: Next, rinse off the food processor bowl. Combine the cream cheese, sugar, and milk in a mixing bowl. Blend until smooth. Then, using a knife, spoon HALF (8 oz) of the Cool Whip into the cream cheese. Fold the mixture with a spatula until it is smooth. Spread the mixture evenly over the crust in the baking dish. Chill.
4. Rinse the food processor bowl once more for the Chocolate Pudding Layer. Combine the chocolate pudding powder, milk, and instant coffee in a mixing bowl. Puree till smooth, covered. In the baking dish, evenly distribute the ingredients.
5. Toppings: Top the chocolate pudding with the remaining 8 oz of Cool Whip. Then, over the top, sprinkle with tiny chocolate chips or chocolate shavings.
6. Place in the refrigerator for at least 4 hours, covered. Freeze for 2-3 hours for optimum cutting results, then cut and serve. Allow 10-15 minutes for the frozen plated pieces to come to room temperature before serving.

Note: This is a fantastic make-ahead dessert that can be made 4-5 days ahead of time and stored in the freezer for up to 3 months.
Nutrition Facts: Calories: 533 | Carbohydrates: 72 g | Protein: 16 g | Fat: 8 g | Cholesterol: 42 mg

188. EASIEST HEALTHY WATERMELON SMOOTHIE RECIPE

Prep Time: 3 minutes
Cook Time: 3 minutes
Total Time: 6 minutes
Servings: 4

Ingredients:
- 4 cups fresh ripe watermelon cubes from a less melon

- 2 cup strawberry yogurt regular or a dairy-free variety
- 4 cups ice
- 1-2 tablespoons granulated sugar optional (Only needed if the watermelon isn't very sweet.)

Directions:
1. In a blender, combine the watermelon cubes and yogurt. Puree till smooth, covered. Taste to see if more sugar is required.
2. Pour in the ice cubes (and sugar if desired). After that, cover and purée until smooth.
3. Serve right away.

Note: Garnish with cubes or slices of watermelon or cut strawberries.

Nutrition Facts: Calories: 120 | Carbohydrates: 27 g | Protein: 27 g | Fat: 19 g | Cholesterol: 47 mg

189. WATERMELON

Prep Time: 5 minutes
Cook Time: 5 minutes
Total Time: 10 minutes
Servings: 4

Ingredients:
- whole watermelon

Directions:
1. Stripes are well defined, with noticeable color differences between the green and yellow lines.
2. A huge yellow patch on the bottom indicates that the watermelon has been ripening on the vine in the field for some time and was not harvested too early.
3. Round versus oblong - Round melons are sweeter than oblong melons. Although most watermelons fall somewhere in the middle, choose a round melon if you have the chance.
4. Weighty is ideal - choose a watermelon that appears to be heavy for its size. This indicates it's jam-packed with juice. Select a few alternatives to compare.
5. Thump the watermelon with a deep tone. The sound should be deep, showing that it is FULL, rather than dried out and airy on the interior.
6. Check the stem - If a stem is connected, it should be dried out and not green. A green stem indicates that the watermelon is in the process of ripening but is not quite ready.
7. Scars and blemishes are desirable - Don't judge a book by its cover. Weathering on the melon's exterior is another sign that it has had plenty of time to sweeten.

Note:
How to cut a watermelon:
Remove the melon's short (stem) ends. Then, from stem end to stem end, cut the watermelon into quarters.
Start at the top of the fruit and cut straight down to the rind in 12 to 1-inch portions for slices.
Then, on each side, cut along the rind's edge, deep into the watermelon to remove the slices from the rind.
To make cubes, cut 1 inch deep into each flat side of the watermelon. Make sure to do this on both sides.
Then, starting at the top, cut down in 1-inch chunks.
Finally, cut along the rind's edge on both sides to release the rind cubes.

Nutrition Facts: Calories: 55 | Carbohydrates: 10 g | Protein: 13 g | Fat: 1 g | Cholesterol: 10 mg

190. BEST ORANGE JULIUS

Prep Time: 5 minutes
Cook Time: 5 minutes
Total Time: 10 minutes
Servings: 3

Ingredients:
- Six oz orange juice concentrate half a can
- One cup of milk 2% or whole
- ½ cup of water
- 1/3 cup granulated sugar
- egg white about 3 tablespoons

- 2 teaspoons of vanilla extract
- ¾ cups ice cubes

Directions:
1. Place all ingredients in the blender.
2. Puree until smooth.

Note:
This Orange Julius copy recipe yields 2 big (20 oz. each) or 4 mini (10 oz.) beverages. Do you want to make a Strawberry or Pineapple Orange Julius? Substitute 8 oz frozen strawberries or frozen pineapple pieces for the orange juice concentrate.

Nutrition Facts: Calories: 179 | Carbohydrates: 36 g | Protein: 4 g | Fat: 1 g | Cholesterol: 6 mg

CHAPTER 9: BREAKFAST (LOW-RESIDUE)

191. CHICKEN VEGETABLE PASTA SOUP

Prep Time: 30 minutes
Cook Time: 30 minutes
Total Time: 60 minutes
Servings: 4

Ingredients:
- 5 cups low sodium chicken broth
- 1 carrot chopped
- 2 potato chopped
- 1/2 cup tomato flesh no skin or s
- 1 bunch of asparagus tips
- 1/2 cup cooked pastini or other small pasta

Directions:
1. In a small saucepan, combine the broth, carrot, and potato. Bring to a boil, then lower to low heat and simmer until the veggies are cooked. Cook until the asparagus is soft, then add the tomatoes and asparagus tips. Cook, constantly stirring, until the pasta is heated through.

Nutrition Facts: Calories: 116 | Carbohydrates: 19 g | Protein: 11 g | Fat: 28 g | Cholesterol: 53 mg

192. BEET CARROT SOUP

Prep Time: 5 minutes
Cook Time: 30 minutes
Total Time: 35 minutes
Servings: 4

Ingredients:
- Four cups of low sodium vegetable broth
- One carrot sliced
- Two can of cooked beets not pickled
- Salt to taste
- non-fat yogurt for serving if desired

Directions:
1. In a small saucepan, combine sliced carrots and vegetable broth. Bring to a boil, then lower to a low heat and continue to simmer, covered, until carrots are very soft. Cook until the beets are cooked through. Puree the soup in a blender until smooth. Season with salt to taste. If preferred, serve with a tablespoon of yogurt mixed in.

Nutrition Facts: Calories: 90 | Carbohydrates: 9 g | Protein: 16 g | Fat: 21 g | Cholesterol: 63 mg

193. BROTH BRAISED ASPARAGUS

Prep Time: 10 minutes
Cook Time: 30 minutes
Total Time: 40 minutes
Servings: 2

Ingredients:
- 1/2 cup of chicken or vegetable broth * check ingredient label carefully if not using homemade broth,
- Two tablespoon olive oil
- For a lemon peel slice, I used a peeler to remove a single slice of lemon.
- 2 cup asparagus tips

Directions:
1. Bring the chicken broth and olive oil to a boil in a saucepan. Combine the lemon peel and asparagus tips in a mixing bowl. Cook for 3-4 minutes, covered, over medium heat, until tender.
2. Before serving, remove the lemon peel.

Note: Only the asparagus tips are acceptable on the Low Residue Diet. The asparagus stalks were saved and cooked separately for the remainder of the family.

Nutrition Facts: Calories: 172 | Carbohydrates: 10 g | Protein: 13 g | Fat: 1 g | Cholesterol: 10 mg

194. LEMON CHICKEN RICE SOUP

Prep Time: 10 minutes
Cook Time: 25 minutes
Total Time: 35 minutes
Servings: 4

Ingredients:
- 2 carrot peeled, chopped
- 1 celery stalk peeled, chopped
- 1/4 cup medium-grain rice such as sushi rice
- 4 cups low sodium chicken broth
- 2 cup cooked chicken breast shredded
- large eggs
- 2 lemon juiced
- 2 cups baby spinach

Directions:
1. In an Instant Pot, combine carrots, celery, rice, and chicken broth. Cook for 10 minutes on high pressure. Allow 15 minutes for natural release before releasing any residual pressure.
2. Remove the lid and turn the Instant Pot to the sauté mode on high. Add the chicken and mix well. Cook until well heated.
3. Combine eggs and lemon juice in a mixing bowl. Whisk in a ladle of hot broth at a time. In a soup pot, whisk together the eggs. Stir in the spinach leaves. Cook until the vegetables are almost soft.

Note Cook the carrots, celery, and rice with a fresh thyme twig in the chicken broth before adding the carrots, celery, and rice.

Nutrition Facts: Calories: 163 | Carbohydrates: 45 g | Protein: 39 g | Fat: 29 g | Cholesterol: 84 mg

195. "MIXED BAG" KALE SALAD

Prep Time: 5 minutes
Cook Time: 5 minutes
Total Time: 10 minutes
Servings: 1

Ingredients:
- Two cups chopped curly kale and in-season mixed greens arugula, baby romaine, red leaf lettuce
- 1/2 cup cherry tomatoes
- 1 ounce shaved gruyere or Parmesan cheese
- Two tablespoons extra virgin olive oil
- Juice from 1/2 lemon

Directions:
1. Toss the kale and other greens, tomatoes, and gruyere cheese together. On top, smear some black. Combine the olive oil and lemon juice. Salad should be dressed before serving.

Nutrition Facts: Calories: 320 | Carbohydrates: 25 g | Protein: 18 g | Fat: 30 g | Cholesterol: 122 mg

196. CHICKEN SAFFRON RICE PILAF

Prep Time: 15 minutes
Cook Time: 25 minutes
Total Time: 40 minutes
Servings: 6

Ingredients:
- Pinch saffron
- tablespoon ghee or olive oil
- One large carrot peeled, chopped
- Two stalk celery outside parts peeled, chopped
- ½ cups of basmati rice or jasmine rice
- 1 cups low sodium chicken broth
- 1/2 teaspoon onion powder
- 1/4 cups poached or roasted chicken breast shredded
- lemon
- fresh parsley chopped

Directions:
1. Soak the saffron in a small dish with a little water.

2. In a large pan, melt the ghee. Sauté carrots and celery for 3-4 minutes, or until carrots soften. Cook until the rice is gently browned and coated with oil.

Cooking in a rice cooker
1. Place rice mixture in a rice cooker. Combine the saffron, chicken broth, and onion powder in a mixing bowl. Set the rice cooker to the white rice option.
2. Toss the rice with the shredded chicken; cover and set aside for 5 minutes until the chicken is cooked through.
3. When ready to serve, pour lemon juice over rice and toss to coat. Garnish with chopped parsley if desired.
4. On the cooktop, I'm preparing a meal.
5. In a pan, combine the saffron, chicken broth, and onion powder. Bring to a boil, then lower heat to medium-low and simmer, covered, for 25-30 minutes, or until tender rice.
6. Toss the rice with the shredded chicken; cover and set aside for 5 minutes until the chicken is cooked through.
7. When ready to serve, pour lemon juice over rice and toss to coat. Garnish with chopped parsley if desired.

Nutrition Facts: Calories: 269 | Carbohydrates: 27 g | Protein: 49 g | Fat: 38 g | Cholesterol: 100 mg

197. VANILLA SOY PUDDING

Prep Time: 5 minutes
Cook Time: 125 minutes
Total Time: 130 minutes
Servings: 4

Ingredients:
- 1/4 ounce unflavored gelatin or powdered agar for a vegan version
- 1/4 cup cold water
- 1/4 cup vanilla soy milk
- 1 cup of tofu
- 1/2 teaspoon vanilla

Directions:

1. Sprinkle gelatin over cold water in a small dish and whisk to dissolve. Allow for a 10-minute rest.
2. Meanwhile, warm the soy milk.
3. Blend the tofu, vanilla, softened gelatin, and heated milk until smooth.
4. Refrigerate until solid, about 2 hours, in four separate containers.

Nutrition Facts: Calories: 105 | Carbohydrates: 18 g | Protein: 63 g | Fat: 5 g | Cholesterol: 89 mg

198. VANILLA PEAR RASPBERRY PANNA COTTA

Prep Time: 10 minutes
Cook Time: 75 minutes
Total Time: 40 minutes
Servings: 6

Ingredients:
- Three cups of cashew milk or other non-dairy milk
- tablespoon unflavored powdered gelatin
- 2 cup low-fat Greek yogurt
- tablespoons honey
- 1/2 teaspoons almond extract

Raspberry Sauce
- 10 oz fresh or frozen raspberries thawed
- 2 tablespoons honey

Poached Pears
- 5 cups unsweetened apple juice
- 1/2 cup orange juice
- vanilla bean or 1 teaspoon vanilla extract
- firm pears peeled

Directions:
1. 1 cup cashew milk in a small dish; sprinkle with unflavored gelatin and stir well; set aside for 3-5 minutes, or until softened.

2. Heat the cashew milk gelatin mixture in a small saucepan over medium heat until the gelatin dissolves (do not let the milk boil). Whisk in the remaining 2 cups of cashew milk, yogurt, honey, and almond extract until completely mixed. Remove from heat and pour into six serving glasses; chill for 5 hours, or until gelled.

Raspberry Sauce
1. In a small saucepan, combine raspberries and honey; simmer, constantly stirring, until raspberries break down, about 4-5 minutes; drain and set raspberry sauce aside until cool.

Poached Pears
1. In a medium saucepan, combine the apple juice and orange juice. Scrape the vanilla beans into the liquid; put the vanilla bean in the saucepan. Bring to a boil; place peeled pears in saucepan; cook for 15 minutes; flip pears over; cook for another 15 minutes, or until a knife easily pokes through. Remove from the fire and set aside to cool; refrigerate the pears in their cooking liquid.

To Serve
1. Remove the panna cotta from the refrigerator and top with a little raspberry sauce. Cut the pear in half lengthwise, leaving the core intact. Using paper towels, drain. Slice the pear halves, leaving approximately 1/2" at the top of each uncut. Place one half on top of each panna cotta.

Nutrition Facts: Calories: 182 | Carbohydrates: 63 g | Protein: 44 g | Fat: 82 g | Cholesterol: 193 mg

199. EGG POTATO BITES

Prep Time: 10 minutes
Cook Time: 25 minutes
Total Time: 35 minutes
Servings: 12

Ingredients:
- Eight large eggs
- One cup low-fat cottage cheese pureed
- sea salt to taste
- Eight oz potato peeled, cooked, chopped
- Two oz swiss cheese or your favorite cheese shredded

Directions:
1. Preheat the oven to 325°F.
2. Coat 12 muffin cups with cooking spray. (Silicone muffin tins are very useful.)
3. Combine the eggs, cottage cheese, and a sprinkle of salt in a mixing bowl. Potatoes should be added. Distribute among the glasses. On top, sprinkle with cheese.
4. Bake for 25-30 minutes, or until the mixture is firm.

Nutrition Facts: Calories: 90 | Carbohydrates: 36 g | Protein: 27 g | Fat: 5 g | Cholesterol: 12 mg

200. BROCCOLI RED EGG BITES

Prep Time: 20 minutes
Cook Time: 15 minutes
Total Time: 35 minutes
Servings: 12

Ingredients:
- 2 tablespoon olive oil
- 1 cups broccoli florets chopped
- 2 cup red bell chopped
- 1 scallion chopped
- 6 large eggs
- sea salt
- black
- 2 teaspoon favorite dried herb blend
- 1 cup low-fat cheddar cheese shredded
- cooking spray

Directions:
1. Preheat the oven to 350°F.
2. In a large skillet, heat the oil. Stir in the broccoli, red bell pepper, and scallions. Season with salt and pepper to taste. Cook for 1-2 minutes. Cover skillet with 1 tablespoon water and simmer until broccoli is barely cooked, approximately another minute or two. Transfer to a platter and set aside to cool to room temperature.

3. Coat nonstick mini muffin pans generously with cooking spray. Divide the cooked veggies among the cans.
4. Combine the eggs, salt, and dry herb mixture in a mixing bowl. Divide the egg mixture among the muffin pans.
5. Place a slice of cheese on top of each pan.
6. Bake for 15 minutes, or until well done.

Nutrition Facts: Calories: 72 | Carbohydrates: 83 g | Protein: 52 g | Fat: 33 g | Cholesterol: 209 mg

201. <u>BREAKFAST SHRIMP EGG WHITE MUFFIN CUPS</u>

Prep Time: 20 minutes
Cook Time: 20 minutes
Total Time: 40 minutes
Servings: 6

Ingredients:
- 2 teaspoons olive oil
- 2 garlic cloves minced
- 3 tablespoon jalapeno finely chopped
- 2 scallion finely chopped
- 1/2 cup red bell sliced or chopped
- 1/4 pound shrimp shelled, deveined, chopped coarsely (~ 3/4 cup)
- 1 cups spinach
- 3 cup plus 2 tablespoons AllWhites 100% liquid egg whites
- 1/8 teaspoon turmeric
- 1/4 teaspoon sea salt
- 1/4 teaspoon black

Directions:
1. Preheat the oven to 375°F.
2. In a large pan, heat the oil and sauté the garlic, jalapeño, white portions of the scallions, red bell pepper, and corn for a minute. Cook for another minute after adding the shrimp, 1/8 teaspoon salt, and 1/8 teaspoon pepper. Sauté the spinach until it is slightly wilted. Remove the pan from the heat and let it cool.
3. Whisk together egg whites, turmeric, 1/8 teaspoon salt, and 1/8 teaspoon in a medium mixing basin.
4. 6 nonstick muffin pans, thoroughly oiled. Divide the shrimp and veggie mixture evenly between the pans. Pour the egg white mixture over the veggies until it reaches the rim of the muffin pans. Top with the green portions of the scallions.
5. Bake for 20 minutes, or until the egg whites are firm.

Nutrition Facts: Calories: 73 | Carbohydrates: 26 g | Protein: 81 g | Fat: 38 g | Cholesterol: 122 mg

202. <u>GARLICKY CHEESY BROCCOLI GRATIN</u>

Prep Time: 15 minutes
Cook Time: 20 minutes
Total Time: 35 minutes
Servings: 4

Ingredients:
- 4 cups organic broccoli trimmed, cut into pieces
- 2 tablespoon olive oil
- 1 small onion minced
- 6 garlic cloves minced, divided
- 1 tablespoon sweet rice flour
- 2 cup low-fat organic milk
- 1/8 teaspoon cayenne
- 1/8 teaspoon ground nutmeg
- 2 tablespoons nutritional yeast
- 3 cup finely shredded sharp free cheddar cheese reserve a few tablespoons for topping
- 1/4 cup gluten-free panko crumbs
- 2 teaspoon dried oregano

Directions:
1. Broccoli should be steamed until barely tender, about 6 minutes; transfer to a baking tray.

2. Heat the oil in a saucepan over medium heat and add the onion and garlic; cook until the onions are cooked, about 3 minutes. Whisk in the rice flour for a minute or two before adding the milk, cayenne pepper, and nutmeg; simmer until slightly thickened. Whisk in the nutritional yeast and shredded cheese until smooth. Season with salt and pepper. Pour the cheese sauce over the steamed broccoli. Combine panko crumbs, oregano, reserved cheddar cheese, salt, and pepper in a mixing bowl. Sprinkle over broccoli-cheese mixture. Broil until the top is gently browned and the cheese has melted.

Nutrition Facts: Calories: 326 | Carbohydrates: 37 g | Protein: 73 g | Fat: 28 g | Cholesterol: 192 mg

203. STEAMED BROCCOLI WITH MISO PEANUT BUTTER SAUCE

Prep Time: 10 minutes
Cook Time: 5 minutes
Total Time: 15 minutes
Servings: 4

Ingredients:
- 2 head broccoli
- Miso Peanut Butter Sauce
- 2 tablespoon light miso
- 1 tablespoon peanut butter
- 2 tablespoon sesame oil
- 4 teaspoon rice vinegar
- 3 teaspoon mirin
- 1-2 tablespoons water to thin sauce

Directions:
Steamed Broccoli
1. Remove the broccoli stem from the broccoli crown. Separate the broccoli head into florets by hand. Trim the broccoli stem and remove the skin. Cut into 1/2-inch pieces. 5-6 minutes, or until barely tender.
2. Sauce with Miso and Peanut Butter

3. Mix all of the ingredients for the Miso Peanut Butter Sauce until well combined. If needed, thin the sauce with extra water.

Nutrition Facts: Calories: 436 | Carbohydrates: 72 g | Protein: 25 g | Fat: 25 g | Cholesterol: 266 mg

204. TOMATO POTATO SAUSAGE PESTO FRITTATA RECIPE

Prep Time: 25 minutes
Cook Time: 30 minutes
Total Time: 55 minutes
Servings: 8

Ingredients:
- 2 tablespoon Garlic Scape Paste or substitute 1 tablespoon olive oil and 2 cloves minced garlic
- 1 large Yukon gold potato peeled, sliced thin
- 1 small onion chopped
- 6 nitrate-free chicken breakfast sausage links cut up
- salt and
- 8 eggs
- 3 tomato chopped
- 1/3 cup shredded jack cheese or cheddar cheese
- 2 tablespoons Kale Mint Basil Pesto
- 1 tablespoons grated Parmesan cheese

Directions:
1. In a large nonstick skillet, heat the Garlic Scape Pesto. Place the potato, onion, and sausage in a pan, cover with 1/2 cup water, and simmer until the potatoes are soft. season with salt and pepper to taste
2. Whisk the eggs in a large mixing dish; add the tomato and jack cheese. Pour the mixture into the skillet. Top with dollops of Kale Mint Basil Pesto. Lift the edges of the frittata with a spatula and tilt the skillet to allow the raw eggs to slip below the frittata.

3. Sprinkle with Parmesan cheese and broil for 2 minutes, or until the top is golden brown.

Nutrition Facts: Calories: 297 | Carbohydrates: 61 g | Protein: 32 g | Fat: 19 g | Cholesterol: 216 mg

205. SKINNY LOADED STUFFED BAKED POTATO SOUP

Prep Time: 20 minutes
Cook Time: 45 minutes
Total Time: 65 minutes
Servings: 5

Ingredients:
- 3 tablespoons extra virgin olive oil, divided
- 2 head cauliflower cut into florets, 1 pound or 4 cups
- 1 small onion chopped, 1/2 cup
- 2 stalk celery chopped, 1/2 cup
- 3 cloves garlic minced
- 4-5 cups low sodium chicken broth
- 1/2 cup raw cashews
- 1/2 teaspoon dried thyme
- 1 medium russet potato peeled, cut into 1/2" pieces
- salt and black to taste

Toppings
- 5 strips turkey bacon
- 5 tablespoons reduced-fat shredded cheddar cheese
- scallion chopped
- 5 tablespoons low-fat Greek yogurt

Directions:
1. Preheat the oven to 375°F. Season cauliflower florets with salt and pepper after tossing with 2 tablespoons olive oil. Place on a baking sheet coated with parchment paper in a single layer. Cook for 20-25 minutes, or until the vegetables are soft and gently browned.
2. In a large saucepan, heat the remaining oil. Combine the onion, celery, and garlic in a mixing bowl. Cook for 2-3 minutes, or until aromatic. Combine 4 cups chicken broth, cashews, thyme, roasted cauliflower, and potatoes in a large mixing bowl. Bring to a boil, then lower to medium-low heat and simmer for 20-25 minutes, or until the potatoes are cooked. As required, add extra chicken broth to cover the veggies.
3. Blend the veggies and soup in a blender until smooth. You may need to perform this in two batches.

Turkey Bacon Bits
1. Mince the turkey bacon finely. Place in a cold skillet and cook over medium heat. Cook, often turning, until the bacon pieces are crisp and browned. Transfer to a plate lined with paper towels.

To Serve
1. Fill serving dishes halfway with blended soup: Turkey bacon pieces, shredded cheese, chopped scallions, and Greek yogurt on top.

Nutrition Facts: Calories: 275 | Carbohydrates: 6 g | Protein: 39 g | Fat: 16 g | Cholesterol: 73 mg

206. SWEET POTATO CASSEROLE WITH PRALINE TOPPING

Prep Time: 20 minutes
Cook Time: 100 minutes
Total Time: 120 minutes
Servings: 8

Ingredients:
- Four pounds of sweet potatoes
- Filling
- Two tablespoons of coconut oil or organic unsalted butter melted
- Two teaspoons of lemon juice
- 1/2 teaspoons vanilla
- Two teaspoons of ground cinnamon
- 1/4 teaspoon ground nutmeg

- 1/8 teaspoon ground cloves
- One teaspoon salt
- 1/4 teaspoon
- One large egg yolks
- Two tablespoons maple syrup
- ¾ cup organic half and half
- Praline Topping
- 1/4 cup gluten-free flour mix
- 1/4 cup organic dark brown sugar
- 2 teaspoon ground cinnamon
- 1/8 teaspoon salt
- ½ tablespoons organic unsalted butter cut into small pieces and softened
- ½ cup of pecans

Directions:
1. Preheat the oven to 400°F. Poke holes in the sweet potatoes with a knife. Place sweet potatoes on a baking sheet coated with foil and roast until they can be squeezed easily (using a kitchen towel and gently squeezing with your hand), about 1 hour or more, depending on the size of the sweet potatoes. Remove from oven and make a longitudinal incision to allow steam to escape. Scoop the meat into a food processor and puree until nearly smooth. Process till mixed the melted coconut oil or butter, lemon juice, vanilla, cinnamon, nutmeg, cloves, salt, egg yolks, and maple syrup. Pour in half and half while the machine is running and process until combined. Spread the mixture into an equal layer in a baking dish. You can cover and refrigerate the dish at this stage until the next day, or you can continue with the Praline Topping.

Praline Topping
1. Preheat the oven to 375°F.
2. In a food processor, mix the flour, brown sugar, cinnamon, and salt. Add butter to a food processor and pulse for a few seconds or until crumbly.
3. Sprinkle the praline topping over the sweet potato mixture—Bake for 40 minutes, or until the topping is nicely browned and the sweet potatoes are heated.

Note: If you don't have dark brown sugar, use 1/4 cup light brown sugar and 1-2 tablespoons molasses instead. It is adapted from a recipe in Cook's Illustrated.
Nutrition Facts: Calories: 400 | Carbohydrates: 66 g | Protein: 17 g | Fat: 15 g | Cholesterol: 137 mg

207. <u>CREAMY GARLIC MASHED CAULIFLOWER AND POTATOES</u>

Prep Time: 10 minutes
Cook Time: 4 minutes
Total Time: 14 minutes
Servings: 4

Ingredients:
- 1/2 cup water chicken or vegetable stock can be used for more flavor
- 2 small head cauliflower or 1/2 large head, core removed
- 1 medium potato peeled
- 2 cloves garlic finely minced
- 2 tablespoons unsalted organic butter
- 2 tablespoons low-fat plain yogurt
- salt and to taste
- minced chives for garnish

Directions:
1. Divide the cauliflower head into quarters.
2. Fill the Instant Pot halfway with water or broth. Place the trivet in the pot. Arrange the potatoes, cauliflower, and garlic on top of the trivet. Cook for 4 minutes on high pressure in a sealed pot. Allow 10-15 minutes for the pressure to dissipate, then remove any residual pressure naturally.
3. Process the cauliflower in a food processor until smooth, scraping down the sides with a spatula as needed.

4. Remove the trivet from the Instant Pot, but leave the broth, garlic, and potatoes in the pot. Blend until smooth (leave a few chunks if you like some texture). To the saucepan, add the pureed cauliflower, butter, and yogurt. Blend until smooth. Season with salt and pepper to taste. Garnish with chives if desired.

Stove Top
1. Cauliflower should be cut into florets. Potatoes should be cut into 1" pieces.
2. Fill a big saucepan halfway with water, just enough to cover the potatoes. Bring the water to a boil. Potatoes should be added. Place the steamer basket over the potatoes, followed by the cauliflower and garlic. Cover and steam the cauliflower for 10 minutes (it should be soft); remove from the heat. Cook for another 10 minutes, covered, until potatoes are soft.
3. Meanwhile, combine the cauliflower and garlic in a food processor and process until smooth, scraping down the sides with a spatula as needed.
4. When the potatoes are cooked, rinse them and mash them until smooth. Combine the cauliflower puree, stock, butter, and yogurt in a mixing bowl. Blend until smooth. Season with salt and pepper. Garnish with chives if desired.

Note: You may need a more or less chicken stock to get the appropriate consistency depending on the size of the cauliflower head and potatoes.

Nutrition Facts: Calories: 182 | Carbohydrates: 38 g | Protein: 47 g | Fat: 31 g | Cholesterol: 140 mg

208. CAULIFLOWER MASHED POTATOES WITH TRUFFLE OIL

Prep Time: 15 minutes
Cook Time: 15 minutes
Total Time: 30 minutes
Servings: 8

Ingredients:
- 2 head organic cauliflower cut into florets
- 5 Yukon gold potatoes peeled, cut into 1/2" slices
- 1/2 cup organic low-fat milk
- 2 tablespoons pastured organic butter
- sea salt
- One tablespoon white truffle oil

Directions:
1. Bring a large saucepan of water to a rolling boil. Cook for 15 minutes, or until the cauliflower and potatoes are soft. Drain thoroughly. In a mixing basin, combine the flour, milk, and butter; beat until smooth. Season with salt and pepper. Drizzle with white truffle oil to finish.

Nutrition Facts: Calories: 122 | Carbohydrates: 37 g | Protein: 47 g | Fat: 39 g | Cholesterol: 323 mg

209. HEALTHY BACON EGG POTATO BREAKFAST CASSEROLE

Prep Time: 20 minutes
Cook Time: 45 minutes
Total Time: 65 minutes
Servings: 9

Ingredients:
- 2 teaspoons olive oil
- 2 medium onion chopped (~ 1 cup)
- 1 red bell chopped (~ 1 cup)
- 3 cup mushrooms chopped
- 2 cloves garlic minced
- 1 strip uncured antibiotic free turkey bacon chopped
- 3 teaspoon Fines Herbes or another herb blend
- 6 large eggs
- 2 cup non-fat cottage cheese pureed in food processor
- 2 cup reduced fat sharp cheddar cheese shredded
- 3 cups shredded Yukon gold potatoes
- 9 cups baby kale

Directions:
1. Preheat the oven to 375°F.
2. In a large pan, heat the oil and sauté the onion, bell pepper, mushrooms, garlic, bacon, and Fines Herbes until the onions are transparent. Place aside.
3. Whisk together the eggs, cottage cheese, and cheddar cheese in a large mixing basin. Mix in the shredded potatoes. Sauté the bacon and veggies. Spoon onto a 9x9 square dish that has been gently oiled.
4. Bake for 45 minutes, or until the casserole is crisp.
5. Serve on top of a bed of young kale.

Nutrition Facts: Calories: 184 | Carbohydrates: 18 g | Protein: 48 g | Fat: 7 g | Cholesterol: 110 mg

210. LEMON-BLUEBERRY MUFFINS

Prep Time: 20 minutes
Cook Time: 0 minutes
Total Time: 20 minutes
Servings: 12

Ingredients:
- 3/4 cup yellow cornmeal
- 3/4 cup whole wheat flour
- 1/2 teaspoons baking powder
- 1/4 cup granulated sugar
- 3/4 cup milk (cow's, soy, or rice)
- 3 tablespoons oil or unsalted butter, melted
- egg, beaten
- 1 tablespoon lemon juice
- 2 teaspoon lemon zest
- 2 cup frozen or fresh blueberries

Directions:
1. Preheat the oven to 400°F.
2. Nonstick cooking spray should be sprayed onto a muffin tray or an 8-inch baking pan.
3. In a large mixing basin, combine cornmeal, flour, baking powder, and sugar.
4. Combine the milk, oil or butter, egg, lemon juice, and lemon zest in a small mixing dish.
5. Stir the milk mixture into the cornmeal mixture until it is barely combined. It is OK to have some lumps.
6. Then, gently fold in the blueberries (if you are using frozen berries, rinse them with cold water and pat dry before adding to the batter).
7. Fill a muffin or 8-inch pan halfway with batter.
8. Bake for 15 minutes if making muffins and 25 minutes if baking in an 8-inch pan.
9. If desired, drizzle with honey.

Nutrition Facts: Calories: 117 | Carbohydrates: 19 g | Protein: 3 g | Fat: 2 g | Cholesterol: 35 mg

211. LEMON-RASPBERRY SAUCE

Prep Time: 5 minutes
Cook Time: 0 minutes
Total Time: 5 minutes
Servings: 6

Ingredients:
- Based on 8 servings per recipe.
- 6 oz frozen raspberries, partially thawed
- 1/4 cup sugar
- 2 tablespoons water
- 2 tablespoon lemon juice

Directions:
1. In a food processor, puree all of the ingredients until smooth. As the sauce sits, it will thicken.

Note: This dish may also be made using strawberries, blackberries, or blueberries. You can alter the sugar to achieve the desired sweetness.

Nutrition Facts: Calories: 28 | Carbohydrates: 4 g | Protein: 1 g | Fat: 1 g | Cholesterol: 17 mg

CHAPTER 10: LUNCH (LOW-RESIDUE)

212. SOUTHERN SHRUB

Prep Time: 10 minutes
Cook Time: 45 minutes
Total Time: 55 minutes
Servings: 6

Ingredients:
- 150 grams fresh or frozen blueberries (if frozen warm to room temperature)
- 200 grams pure honey
- 250 ml white vinegar
- 2 liter soda water or mineral water
- 1 star fruit for decoration
- 2 mint leaves for decoration

Directions:
1. Fill a big heatproof jar halfway with blueberries.
2. Bring honey and vinegar to a boil in a heavy-bottomed pot and whisk to combine all ingredients.
3. Pour the mixture over the berries and mash them down with a potato masher or fork (whatever fits in the jar) to extract the juice.
4. Store the glass jar in a cool area for 3 days.
5. Chill the mixture for a week in the fridge after straining it through muslin or fine cheesecloth into a transparent container.
6. When ready to serve, fill a tall glass with ice, 1/3 blueberry juice, then gently top with sparkling water for a two-tone effect.
7. Garnish the glass with a thick slice of star fruit on the side and a mint leaf on top.

Nutrition Facts: Calories: 246 | Carbohydrates: 9 g | Protein: 18 g | Fat: 11 g | Cholesterol: 27 mg

213. ROSEMARY LIME KISS

Prep Time: 10 minutes
Cook Time: 5 minutes
Total Time: 15 minutes
Servings: 4

Ingredients:
- One big grapefruit (or 1 large grapefruit and 12 blood or regular orange juice) 200 mL freshly squeezed ruby grapefruit juice
- 300 ml sparkling mineral water
- Thin wedges of blood orange for decoration
- Spiral peel two limes
- Two juiced of limes
- If you want a sweeter flavor, use stevia drops.
- Two stems of rosemary leaves

Directions:
1. 10 minutes to chill two tall glasses
2. Pour two limes and two freshly squeezed red grapefruit into a water jug. sweeten to taste with stevia
3. Remove cooled glasses from the refrigerator.
4. Fill glasses with ice.
5. Pour the mixture into the cooled glasses over the ice.
6. Each glass should have a spiraled lime peel and a stem of rosemary.
7. To produce a two-tone appearance, gently top with sparkling water.
8. Serve with an orange slice on the side of the glass.

Nutrition Facts: Calories: 172 | Carbohydrates: 39 g | Protein: 47 g | Fat: 38 g | Cholesterol: 192 mg

214. RUBY RED PUNCH

Prep Time: 5 minutes
Cook Time: 10 minutes
Total Time: 15 minutes
Servings: 6

Ingredients:
- 250 grams frozen strawberries
- 2 fresh strawberries halved for decoration

- 4 finely chopped mint leaves for decoration
- 120 ml organic coconut water
- 2 cups ice
- 2 small less watermelon
- 1 fresh lemon juiced
- 2 Stevia drops if you like a sweeter taste

Directions:
1. Watermelon should be cut in half and the flesh scooped out with an ice cream scoop or spoon and placed in a blender.
2. Squeeze three lemons into a bowl. Blend in a blender with frozen *strawberries and coconut water.
3. It can be refrigerated for a few hours.
4. To serve, combine the juice and two cups of ice in a blender and mix until smooth.
5. Serve immediately in a chilled martini glass, garnished with a half heart-shaped strawberry and a sprinkle of shredded mint.

Nutrition Facts: Calories: 55 | Carbohydrates: 10 g | Protein: 13 g | Fat: 1 g | Cholesterol: 10 mg

215. EGGY DEVILS

Prep Time: 10 minutes
Cook Time: 20 minutes
Total Time: 30 minutes
Servings: 12

Ingredients:
- 3 tablespoons whole egg organic mayonnaise
- 6 free range eggs
- Pinch of turmeric powder
- Pinch of mustard powder
- Salt and to taste
- Paprika to dust eggs with
- A packet of water crackers

Directions:
1. In a saucepan, combine the eggs, cover with water, and heat. Allow the eggs to simmer for 4 12 minutes after they have reached a boil.
2. Remove the eggs from the heat and immerse them in cold water for one minute before carefully peeling and slicing them half lengthwise.
3. Scoop the yolks into a mixing dish and mash with the mayonnaise, turmeric, mustard, and salt & pepper to taste.
4. Remove a small slice from the rounded bottom of the egg white halves to ensure they rest securely on the plate or cracker, then pipe or spoon the yolk mixture back into the white egg halves.
5. Serve with a little dusting of paprika on top.

Nutrition Facts: Calories: 182 | Carbohydrates: 43 g | Protein: 37 g | Fat: 40 g | Cholesterol: 61 mg

216. CARAMEL SAUCED ORANGES

Prep Time: 10 minutes
Cook Time: 15 minutes
Total Time: 25 minutes
Servings: 4

Ingredients:
- 4 large oranges
- 1 juiced orange
- 1/2 cup brown demerara sugar
- 1/4 cup water
- 2 teaspoon allspice

Directions:
1. Peel the oranges, removing the white portion, then segment the oranges to remove the majority of the membrane, leaving only the meat.
2. Each section should be cut in half.
3. Place the orange juice, allspice, sugar, and water in a heavy bottomed pan.
4. Bring to a boil over medium heat for 5-10 minutes, or until the mixture turns caramel slightly in color and thickens.
5. Arrange the orange segments on each of the four dishes and pour the caramel over each.

6. Serve with vanilla yogurt, coconut yogurt, or ice cream.

Nutrition Facts: Calories: 271 | Carbohydrates: 22 g | Protein: 73 g | Fat: 12 g | Cholesterol: 88 mg

217. PULLED CHICKEN SALAD

Prep Time: 20 minutes
Cook Time: 30 minutes
Total Time: 50 minutes
Servings: 4

Ingredients:
- 200 grams cooked pulled BBQ chicken
- 1/3 cup drained tinned apricots thinly sliced
- 100 grams dry weight of orzo pasta
- 150 grams baby spinach with stalks removed
- 70 grams fontina cheese (or cheddar) cut into small cubes
- 30 grams parmesan cheese
- 1/4 cup finely chopped parsley
- 1/3 cup Chang's ® fried noodles
- 5 tablespoon olive oil
- 3 tablespoon red wine vinegar
- salt and to taste

Directions:
1. With a fork, shred cooked and chilled chicken.
2. Place cooked, cooled orzo pasta in a microwave-safe dish, stir in fontina and parmesan cheese, and microwave for 1-2 minutes, or until the cheese is just melted, then mix through the pasta.
3. Allow the salad to cool before adding the spinach, parsley, chicken, and apricots.
4. Combine the olive oil, red wine vinegar, and salt in a mixing bowl and drizzle over the salad. Mix thoroughly.
5. To keep the crispy noodles crunchy, add them right before serving.
6. Serve alone or with crusty white Ciabatta and an olive oil dip.

Nutrition Facts: Calories: 200 | Carbohydrates: 18 g | Protein: 11 g | Fat: 26 g | Cholesterol: 380 mg

218. BEETROOT CARROT SALAD

Prep Time: 10 minutes
Cook Time: 20 minutes
Total Time: 30 minutes
Servings: 4

Ingredients:
- 3 golden beetroots (peeled) or 3 large carrots (skin left on) or a mixture of both
- 500 grams halloumi (thickly sliced)
- 2 teaspoon fresh oregano leaves
- 100 ml maple syrup
- 50 ml fresh lemon juice
- 50 grams spinach leaves
- 200 grams hulled tahini
- 100 grams Chang's crispy noodles
- 1 tablespoon extra virgin olive oil

Directions:
1. Preheat the oven to 180°C for 10 minutes. Wrap the beets and/or carrots in foil and bake for 40 minutes, or until tender. Allow cooling before cutting into wedges.
2. Heat the olive oil in a saucepan over medium heat and brown the halloumi on both sides.
3. Reduce the heat to low and whisk in the maple syrup, lemon juice, and oregano.
4. Spread a tablespoon of hulled tahini and a few baby spinach leaves, then top with the haloumi and beet/carrot wedges on each serving dish.
5. Top with crispy noodles and any remaining liquid.

Nutrition Facts: Calories: 172 | Carbohydrates: 18 g | Protein: 37 g | Fat: 54 g | Cholesterol: 38 mg

219. LEMONGRASS BEEF

Prep Time: 20 minutes
Cook Time: 45 minutes
Total Time: 65 minutes
Servings: 4

Ingredients:
- 2 tablespoons oil
- 1 tablespoon fish sauce
- 2 tablespoons sweet chili sauce
- 2 packets microwave basmati rice
- 2 teaspoons shredded coconut
- 1 tablespoon lemongrass paste
- 500 grams lean grass-fed beef mince
- 3 tube or tub Gourmet Thai seasoning stir in paste
- 100 grams of peeled Lebanese cucumber cut into chunks
- 2 carrots peeled and julienned
- 1/4 cup chopped Thai basil (for decorating)
- 2 lime cut into 4 to serve.

Directions:
1. Heat the oil in a wok and add the Thai seasoning, fish sauce, lemongrass paste, and Thai seasoning. Stir rapidly before adding the minced meat.
2. 3-4 minutes, or until browned.
3. Heat the ready-to-eat rice according to the package directions.
4. When ready, mix in a teaspoon of shredded coconut to each packet, taking caution not to burn yourself with the hot steam.
5. Combine the mince, rice, cucumber, and carrots in a mixing bowl, then top with the Thai basil and a dab of sweet chili sauce.
6. Serve with a quarter of a lime.

Nutrition Facts: Calories: 122 | Carbohydrates: 19 g | Protein: 16 g | Fat: 38 g | Cholesterol: 25 mg

220. MANGO PRAWN POKE BOWL

Prep Time: 20 minutes
Cook Time: 20 minutes
Total Time: 40 minutes
Servings: 6

Ingredients:
- 2 large avocado cut into chunks
- 1 mango cut into chunks
- ½ cups white basmati rice
- 6 tablespoons peeled shredded carrot
- 400 grams cooked prawns chopped into small bites
- 50 grams spinach leaves
- 1/2 cup finely chopped parsley

Dressing
- 2 teaspoon lemongrass pulp
- 3 teaspoon powdered garlic
- 60 ml extra virgin olive oil
- 50 ml fresh lime juice
- salt and to taste

Directions:
1. Separately place the white rice, mango pieces, avocado, shredded carrot, prawns (or tofu), baby spinach leaves in each bowl, then top with chopped parsley.
2. Add the dressing ingredients to a clean container, tightly shut the lid, and shake well to combine. Pour an even quantity over the contents in each bowl.

Nutrition Facts: Calories: 182 | Carbohydrates: 22 g | Protein: 13 g | Fat: 4 g | Cholesterol: 77 mg

221. CITRUS SWORDFISH

Prep Time: 30 minutes
Cook Time: 30 minutes
Total Time: 60 minutes
Servings: 2

Ingredients:
- Two swordfish steaks (about 3/4-inch thick) (about 6 oz each).

- Grated citrus zest (lemon, orange, and lime) (approximately Two tablespoons total; to get the zest, finely grate the peel of whole fruit, being careful not to include bitter white skin).
- Two tablespoons fresh parsley, chopped
- Three tablespoons fresh thyme, chopped
- Three teaspoon olive oil

Directions:
1. Preheat the broiler. Combine the zest, herbs, and oil in a mixing bowl. Place the steaks in a flat pan and brush with the zest mixture on both sides. Broil the fish for 3 to 4 minutes. Broil for 3 to 4 minutes, or until done. Pour pan juices over swordfish and serve immediately, topped with orange, lemon, and lime slices.

Nutrition Facts: Calories: 232 | Carbohydrates: 34 g | Protein: 9 g | Fat: 15 g | Cholesterol: 63 mg

222. **HONEY-HERB CHICKEN**

Prep Time: 30 minutes
Cook Time: 60 minutes
Total Time: 90 minutes
Servings: 4

Ingredients:
- 4 boneless, skinless chicken breast halves (about 1 pound)
- Juice of 1 lime (about 2 tablespoons)
- 2 tablespoons fresh coriander, chopped
- 2 tablespoon honey

Directions:
1. Pound each breast half to approximately 1/2-inch thick with a meat tenderizer. In a small bowl, combine the lime juice, coriander, and honey. Brush the glaze over the chicken breasts. Brush the grill with olive oil. Grill (or broil) the chicken for 5 minutes on each side, or until it reaches an internal temperature of 165°F. It can be served immediately or refrigerated for later use in sandwiches or salads.

Nutrition Facts: Calories: 149 | Carbohydrates: 28 g | Protein: 13 g | Fat: 1 g | Cholesterol: 10 mg

223. **RED ROSEMARY VINEGAR**

Prep Time: 20 minutes
Cook Time: 15 minutes
Total Time: 35 minutes
Servings: 4

Ingredients:
- 3 quart red wine vinegar
- 2 handful rosemary sprigs
- 2 thoroughly clean 16-ounce jars with plastic lids

Directions:
1. Rinse and dry the rosemary. Lightly crush to release the aroma, then split into two jars. Pour vinegar into a nonreactive pan (nearly anything except metal) and bring to a boil (about 8 to 10 minutes at medium-high heat). Fill jars with vinegar and cover with lids. Allow for a two-week rest period.
2. Pour vinegar into beautiful bottles to make a present. Fill the new bottle with a fresh sprig of rosemary. Seal and present the document.
3. The acidity of vinegar makes it safer than other home-canning ventures. However, if your flavored vinegar begins to mold or shows indications of fermentation (bubbling, severe cloudiness, or sliminess), discard it!

Nutrition Facts: Calories: 182 | Carbohydrates: 22 g | Protein: 19 g | Fat: 36 g | Cholesterol: 28 mg

224. **HERB-CRUSTED TILAPIA**

Prep Time: 20 minutes
Cook Time: 60 minutes
Total Time: 80 minutes
Servings: 4

Ingredients:

- 2 tilapia fillets (about 3/4 pound)
- 2 tablespoon flour
- 2 large eggs, plus 1 tablespoon water
- tablespoons mixed herbs
- 1/2 cup panko (Japanese-style breadcrumbs)
- 2 tablespoons of olive oil

Directions:
1. Flour should be sprinkled on waxed paper. Flour should be rubbed into the fillets. In a small bowl, whisk together the egg and the water. Combine panko and herbs on waxed paper. Dip the floured fillets in the egg wash, roll in the herb-panko mixture, and pat it lightly to adhere to the fish. In a nonstick frying pan, heat the oil to medium high. Cook the salmon for around 3 minutes. Cook for another 3 minutes, turning once. Serve right away.

Nutrition Facts: Calories: 317 | Carbohydrates: 39 g | Protein: 28 g | Fat: 28 g | Cholesterol: 182 mg

225. STIR-FRY VELVETED CHICKEN AND VEGETABLES

Prep Time: 25 minutes
Cook Time: 30 minutes
Total Time: 55 minutes
Servings: 4

Ingredients:
- Velveted Chicken
- Three pound boneless skinless chicken breast
- 1/2 teaspoon salt
- Three tablespoon rice wine
- Three large egg white
- Two tablespoon cornstarch
- Three tablespoons oil
- Vegetables
- Two cups chicken broth or water
- Two carrots peeled, cut into 1/2" thick slices
- Three shitake mushrooms stem removed, quartered
- Three medium zucchini peeled, s scooped out, sliced into 1/2" thick slices
- Two bunch asparagus tips
- Stir-Fry Sauce
- Two tablespoons of soy sauce
- Two tablespoons of oyster sauce
- One tablespoon of rice wine
- 1/2 teaspoon sugar
- Two teaspoons of cornstarch dissolved in 2 tablespoons cold water
- Three teaspoons oil
- Stir-Fry
- 2 teaspoons oil
- 3 slice ginger peeled, finely minced
- ¼ cup low sodium chicken stock

Directions:
Velveting Chicken
1. Chicken should be cut into thin slices, tiny cubes, or thin strips. Add salt and rice wine to a mixing bowl and stir thoroughly. With a fork, whisk the egg white until the gel is broken down. Mix in the cornstarch and add to the chicken. Stir in 1 tablespoon of oil until thoroughly combined. Refrigerate for at least 30 minutes, covered.
2. 1 quart of water, brought to a boil Reduce the heat to low and add 1 tablespoon oil. Stir the chicken into the saucepan to separate the pieces. Continue to whisk until the coating becomes white. Then strain quickly in a colander.

Cooking Vegetables
1. In a saucepan, bring chicken broth to a boil. Toss in the carrot slices. Cook until the vegetables are soft. Using a slotted spoon, remove from pan.
2. Cook until the mushrooms and zucchini are soft in the chicken stock. Using a slotted spoon, remove from pan. Cook until the asparagus tips are tender in the pan. Using a slotted spoon, remove from pan. Reserve 1/4 of the chicken stock for the stir-fry; save the rest for another use.

Stir-Fry Sauce
1. Stir together the Stir-Fry Sauce ingredients in a small dish.
2. Chicken with Vegetables in a Stir-Fry

3. In a wok or big pan, heat the oil. Stir in the ginger for a few seconds or until it's aromatic. Cooked veggies should be added to the wok. Serve with velveted chicken on top. Cover the wok with 1/4 cup chicken stock. Cook for 1 minute on high.

4. Stir in the Stir-Fry Sauce and mix for 1 minute to coat the chicken and veggies with the sauce. Serve.

Nutrition Facts: Calories: 315 | Carbohydrates: 19 g | Protein: 14 g | Fat: 14 g | Cholesterol: 73 mg

CHAPTER 11: DINNER (LOW-RESIDUE)

226. BACON & BALSAMIC TOMATOES

Prep Time: 10 minutes
Cook Time: 20 minutes
Total Time: 30 minutes
Servings: 4

Ingredients:
- 4 center-cut bacon strips, chopped
- 4 cod fillets (5 oz each)
- 1/2 teaspoon salt
- 1/4 teaspoon
- 2 cups grape tomatoes, halved
- 2 tablespoons balsamic vinegar

Directions:
1. Cook bacon in a large pan over medium heat until crisp, turning regularly. Drain on paper towels after removing with a slotted spoon.
2. Season the fillets with salt and pepper. Cook until the fish just begins to flake easily with a fork, 4-6 minutes on each side, in the bacon drippings. Take out and keep warm.
3. Cook and stir until the tomatoes are softened, about 2-4 minutes. Reduce the heat to medium-low after stirring in the vinegar. Cook until the sauce thickens, about 1-2 minutes more. Serve the fish with the tomato-bacon combination.

Nutrition Facts: Calories: 55 | Carbohydrates: 25 g | Protein: 26 g | Fat: 9 g | Cholesterol: 28 mg

227. CHOCOLATE-CHIPOTLE SIRLOIN STEAK

Prep Time: 10 minutes
Cook Time: 20 minutes
Total Time: 30 minutes
Servings: 4

Ingredients:
- 3 tablespoons baking cocoa
- 2 tablespoons chopped chipotles in adobo sauce
- 4 teaspoons Worcestershire sauce
- 2 teaspoons brown sugar
- 1/2 teaspoon salt
- 1-1/2 pounds beef top sirloin steak

Directions:
1. In a blender, combine the first 5 ingredients; cover and process until smooth. Rub over the beef. Refrigerate for at least 2 hours, covered.
2. Grill beef, covered, over medium heat for 8-10 minutes on each side, or until meat reaches desired doneness (a thermometer should register 135° for medium-rare, 140° for medium, and 145° for medium-well).

Nutrition Facts: Calories: 246 | Carbohydrates: 6 g | Protein: 37 g | Fat: 6 g | Cholesterol: 17 mg

228. CHEESE SAUCE

Prep Time: 5 minutes
Cook Time: 10 minutes
Total Time: 15 minutes
Servings: 4

Ingredients:
- ¼ Cup Butter
- ¼ Cup Cream Cheese
- ½ Cup Heavy Whipping Cream
- Two Cups of Cheddar Cheese

Directions:
1. Melt the butter over medium heat. Then stir in the cream cheese. Stir until the cream cheese is completely melted. Slowly pour in the heavy cream, constantly stirring until the mixture comes to a boil.
2. Stir in the cheddar cheese until it is thoroughly mixed. Allow to boil for 5-10 minutes over low heat, or until the desired thickness is attained.

Nutrition Facts: Calories: 369 | Carbohydrates: 7 g | Protein: 30 g | Fat: 25 g | Cholesterol: 182 mg

229. CROCKPOT CREAM CHEESE CHICKEN

Prep Time: 5 minutes
Cook Time: 510 minutes
Total Time: 515 minutes
Servings: 6

Ingredients:
- 3 Pkg Cream cheese
- 3 Pckt Italian dressing seasoning
- Chicken Breast
- 2 Can Cream of Chicken Soup

Directions:
1. Coat your crockpot with nonstick cooking spray.
2. Put your chicken breasts in there.
3. Place the cream cheese and chicken cream on top of the chicken breasts.
4. Season the ingredients using the package of Italian dressing seasoning.
5. Cook for 6-8 hours on low heat (I stirred halfway through to make sure it was all mixed up)
6. Serve alongside rice or spaghetti.

Nutrition Facts: Calories: 174 | Carbohydrates: 7 g | Protein: 10 g | Fat: 4 g | Cholesterol: 186 mg

230. 2 MINUTE FLOURLESS ENGLISH MUFFIN

Prep Time: 1 minute
Cook Time: 2 minutes
Total Time: 3 minutes
Servings: 1

Ingredients:
- 1/3 cup rolled oats gluten free, if necessary- For PALEO/GRAIN FREE option, see link above
- 3 tablespoon chia
- ½ teaspoon baking powder
- 2 tablespoon unsweetened applesauce
- 2 tablespoon milk of choice
- Optional: a pinch of salt

Directions:
1. Combine the oats, chia seeds, baking powder, and salt in a blender. Blend on high until the mixture is finely ground.
2. Transfer to a mixing dish and stir in the applesauce and non-dairy milk to make a sticky dough.
3. Place the dough in a ramekin and press it down.
4. Microwave on high for 2 minutes.
5. Allow it to cool for 5 minutes before taking it from the ramekin.
6. Cut in half, toast, and serve with desired toppings.

Nutrition Facts: Calories: 174 | Carbohydrates: 22 g | Protein: 7 g | Fat: 6 g | Cholesterol: 19 mg

231. POTATOES RECIPE

Prep Time: 5 minutes
Cook Time: 5 minutes
Total Time: 10 minutes
Servings: 4

Ingredients:
- 2 head cauliflower
- 2 cup water
- ¼ cup sour cream
- ⅓ cup mayonnaise more or less as desired
- salt and to taste
- Parsley for garnish

Directions:
1. Remove the cauliflower florets from the stalk and split or chop them into bite-size pieces.
2. Fill the instant pot halfway with water and place the cauliflower florets on a trivet (some may fall through).
3. Cover with a lid and turn the toggle switch to the sealing position.
4. For 5 minutes, press "Manual."

5. When the cooking is finished, allow the steam to naturally escape for 10 minutes before releasing it by flipping the toggle switch to the "venting" position.
6. Place the cauliflower in a mixing dish with sour cream, mayonnaise, salt, and pepper.
7. Use a potato masher to mash and combine, and an immersion blender for a smoother consistency.
8. Adjust the salt and pepper to taste. Garnish with parsley and serve right away.
9. Enjoy!

Nutrition Facts: Calories: 190 | Carbohydrates: 7 g | Protein: 3 g | Fat: 17 g | Cholesterol: 15 mg

232. <u>PEANUT BUTTER AND JELLY PB&J SMOOTHIE</u>

Prep Time: 5 minutes
Cook Time: 0 minutes
Total Time: 5 minutes
Servings: 2

Ingredients:
- cup froze mixed berries
- tablespoons peanut butter powder (get it here)
- scoop dairy free vanilla protein powder (about 30g)
- ½ cups almond milk or coconut milk

Directions:
1. In a blender, combine all of the ingredients and pulse until smooth and creamy.

Nutrition Facts: Calories: 140 | Carbohydrates: 10 g | Protein: 13 g | Fat: 27 g | Cholesterol: 188 mg

233. <u>CHOCOLATE MASON JAR ICE CREAM</u>

Prep Time: 8 minutes
Cook Time: 10 minutes
Total Time: 18 minutes
Servings: 4

Ingredients:
- cup heavy cream
- tablespoons granular monk fruit
- tablespoon unsweetened cocoa powder
- teaspoon pure vanilla extract
- tablespoons sugar free chocolate chips, optional

Directions:
1. In a wide opening pint sized mason jar, combine all of the ingredients. Screw on the lid and vigorously shake for 5 minutes. The liquid in the side should have doubled in volume, filling the mason jar.
2. Freeze for at least 3 hours and up to 24 hours.
3. Scoop and savor!

Nutrition Facts: Calories: 206 | Carbohydrates: 1 g | Protein: 18 g | Fat: 1 g | Cholesterol: 26 mg

234. <u>DRY RUB RIBS</u>

Prep Time: 20 minutes
Cook Time: 150 minutes
Total Time: 170 minutes
Servings: 6

Ingredients:
- 2 pounds pork baby back ribs
- 2 tablespoons olive oil
- 2 batch Barbecue Dry Rub

Directions:
1. Preheat the oven to 300 degrees Fahrenheit. Aluminum foil should be used to line a rimmed baking pan.
2. Remove the thin membrane from the ribs' rear, or concave side. Begin by slicing the membrane with a sharp knife and pulling the skin away from the ribs. Place the ribs on a baking sheet that has been lined with parchment paper.

3. Brush the ribs equally with olive oil. Spread the dry rub evenly over both sides of the ribs.
4. Bake for approximately 2 12 hours, or until the ribs are tender and juicy on the inside and beautiful and crispy on the exterior. Refrigerate any leftovers for up to a week.

Nutrition Facts: Calories: 400 | Carbohydrates: 3 g | Protein: 43 g | Fat: 17 g | Cholesterol: 73 mg

235. PROSCIUTTO & SPINACH EGG CUPS

Prep Time: 15 minutes
Cook Time: 30 minutes
Total Time: 45 minutes
Servings: 6

Ingredients:
- 6 slices prosciutto
- 6 eggs
- 1/2 cup baby spinach
- 1/4 tablespoon, salt optional

Directions:
1. Preheat the Air Fryer or Oven to 375°F.
2. While it preheats, place one slice of prosciutto in each cup, pushing it down to line the bottom and edges.
3. As long when your muffin pan is recent, you don't need to spray it first; as the prosciutto cooks, it will naturally come away from the tin if you're unsure, spritz or sprinkle a little oil inside first.
4. Press approximately 4-5 spinach leaves into the bottom of each cup.
5. Each cup should have one egg. Then sprinkle with a bit more and they're ready to bake or cook in the air fryer.
6. In the Air Fryer, bake. Close the air fryer after carefully transferring your muffin tray or cups (leave a little space between them). The cooking time is 10 minutes.
7. Bake in the oven: Place the silicone muffin cups on a baking sheet. Place the muffin tin or baking sheet on the center rack of the oven and bake for 15 minutes for a medium cooked egg.

Nutrition Facts: Calories: 97 | Carbohydrates: 1 g | Protein: 7 g | Fat: 2 g | Cholesterol: 169 mg

CHAPTER 12: BREAKFAST (FIBER-RICH)

236. HIGH-FIBRE MUESLI

Prep Time: 5 minutes
Cook Time: 15 minutes
Total Time: 20 minutes
Servings: 4

Ingredients:
- 300g jumbo oats
- 100g All-Bran
- 25g wheatgerm
- 100g dark raisins
- 140g ready-to-eat apricots, snipped into chunks
- 50g golden lin

Directions:
1. In a large mixing basin, combine all of the ingredients. In an airtight container, this can be stored for up to 2 months. When you're ready to serve, pour in a generous amount of cold milk and let it soak for a few minutes.

Nutrition Facts: Calories: 125 | Carbohydrates: 23 g | Protein: 46 g | Fat: 4 g | Cholesterol: 73 mg

237. MEXICAN BEAN SOUP WITH GUACAMOLE

Prep Time: 10 minutes
Cook Time: 20 minutes
Total Time: 30 minutes
Servings: 2

Ingredients:
- 2 tablespoon rape oil
- 2 large onions, finely chopped
- 1 red, cut into chunks
- 2 garlic cloves, chopped
- 3 tablespoon mild chili powder
- 5 tablespoon ground coriander
- 3 tablespoon ground cumin
- 400g can chopped tomatoes
- 400g can black beans
- 2 tablespoon vegetable bouillon powder
- 3 small avocado
- handful chopped coriander
- 2 lime, juiced
- ½ red chili, deed and finely chopped (optional)

Directions:
1. In a medium skillet, heat the oil, add the onion (reserving 1 tablespoon to prepare the guacamole later), and cook for 10 minutes, stirring constantly. Stir in the garlic and spices, then add the tomatoes, beans, liquid, half a can of water, and bouillon powder. Cook, covered, for 15 minutes.
2. Meanwhile, peel and de-stone the avocado and place it in a mixing bowl with the remaining onion, coriander, and lime juice, as well as a pinch of chili (if using), and mash thoroughly. Serve the soup in two dishes, topped with guacamole.

Nutrition Facts: Calories: 391 | Carbohydrates: 15 g | Protein: 2 g | Fat: 11 g | Cholesterol: 120 mg

238. WHOLEMEAL SODA BREAD

Prep Time: 10 minutes
Cook Time: 25 minutes
Total Time: 35 minutes
Servings: 4

Ingredients:
- 450g wholemeal flour, plus extra for dusting
- 75g four- mix (sunflower, golden lin and pumpkin)
- 3 tablespoon bicarbonate of soda
- 3 tablespoon black treacle
- 150ml pot natural bio yogurt made up to 450ml with water

Directions:

3. Preheat the oven to 200°C/180°C fan/gas 6 and line a baking sheet with parchment paper. In a large mixing basin, combine the flour, s, bicarbonate of soda, and a pinch of salt. When the treacle has dissolved in the yogurt mixture, pour it over the dry ingredients. Stir everything together with a knife until you have a moist, sticky dough. Allow for 5 minutes (this allows time for the liquid to absorb into the bran).
4. Form the dough into a circle approximately 18cm wide on a lightly floured board. It will still be extremely sticky, so don't overwork it; treat it more like scone dough than bread dough. Bake for 25-30 minutes, or until the crust is brown and the loaf sounds hollow when tapped beneath.

Nutrition Facts: Calories: 183 | Carbohydrates: 27 g | Protein: 71 g | Fat: 3 g | Cholesterol: 162 mg

239. SCRAMBLED EGGS

Prep Time: 10 minutes
Cook Time: 15 minutes
Total Time: 25 minutes
Servings: 2

Ingredients:
- block firm tofu (12.3 oz)
- 1/2 head red onion
- 2 stem scallion
- 1/2 head bell
- 5-6 fresh basil leaves
- 1/2 cup oat milk
- 3 tablespoon nutritional yeast
- 1/3 tablespoon turmeric
- tablespoon salt
- 1/3 tablespoon black salt *optional

Directions:
1. Scramble the tofu block with your hands into little and larger bits (as seen in the photo above).
2. In a pan, heat 1 tablespoon of oil over medium heat. Make a caramel sauce with chopped red onions.
3. Stir in the scrambled tofu for 1 minute.
4. Stir in the 1/2 cup oat milk until the tofu has absorbed most of it.
5. When there is just a tiny quantity of milk left, add the other ingredients and whisk for 3-4 minutes on low to medium heat.
6. Serve with warm bread.

Nutrition Facts: Calories: 246 | Carbohydrates: 9 g | Protein: 15 g | Fat: 15 g | Cholesterol: 66 mg

240. STRAWBERRY BREAKFAST CAKE

Prep Time: 15 minutes
Cook Time: 30 minutes
Total Time: 45 minutes
Servings: 15

Ingredients:
- Breakfast Cake
- 2 cups oat flour
- 3 cup almond flour
- 4 tablespoon chia
- 2 teaspoons baking powder
- 1/2 teaspoon salt
- 1/2 cup maple syrup
- 1/2 cup almond milk
- 2 teaspoon vanilla
- 1/2 teaspoon almond extract
- 2 teaspoon grated lemon zest
- 1 cup strawberries, hulled and roughly chopped

Frosting
- 3 cup cashews, soaked for 2 hours
- 1/3 cup maple syrup
- 1/4 cup almond milk
- 1/2 cup strawberries, diced (divided in half)
- 3 teaspoon vanilla extract
- 2 teaspoon lemon juice

Directions:
For Cake
1. Preheat the oven to 350°F. Set aside an 8x8 baking sheet lined with parchment paper and gently greased.

2. Combine oat flour, almond flour, chia seeds, baking powder, and salt in a large mixing basin.
3. Stir in the maple syrup, almond milk, vanilla, almond extract, and lemon zest until thoroughly mixed. Finally, fold in the strawberries.
4. Bake for 40 minutes, or until a fork inserted into the center of the cake comes out clean.
5. Allow cooling fully before adding the icing!

Frosting

6. Drain and rinse cashews before adding to a blender (preferably high-speed). Pour in the maple syrup, almond milk, 1/4 cup strawberries, vanilla essence, and lemon juice.
7. Blend on and off, stopping to scrape the frosting down the sides of the blender until the frosting is smooth and creamy, about 5 minutes.
8. Stir in the remaining fresh chopped strawberries in a basin. Refrigerate until ready to serve or serve right away.

Nutrition Facts: Calories: 171 | Carbohydrates: 25 g | Protein: 13 g | Fat: 7 g | Cholesterol: 19 mg

241. BLUEBERRY PROTEIN SHAKE

Prep Time: 5 minutes
Cook Time: 5 minutes
Total Time: 10 minutes
Servings: 2

Ingredients:
- scoop vanilla protein powder
- 8 oz unsweetened almond milk
- 1/2 cup blueberries fresh or frozen
- Two cups of ice

Directions:
1. In a blender, combine all of the ingredients and mix until smooth.
2. If the smoothie is too thick, add additional almond milk and re-blend.
3. If the smoothie is too thin, add more ice and mix once more.

Nutrition Facts: Calories: 520 | Carbohydrates: 43 g | Protein: 18 g | Fat: 19 g | Cholesterol: 272 mg

242. CHICKPEA SCRAMBLE BREAKFAST BOWL

Prep Time: 10 minutes
Cook Time: 10 minutes
Total Time: 20 minutes
Servings: 2

Ingredients:
Chickpea Scramble
- 15 oz Can of Chickpeas
- 1/2 Tablespoon Turmeric
- 1/2 Tablespoon Salt
- 1/2 Tablespoon
- 1/4 White Onion diced
- 2 Cloves Garlic minced
- Drizzle Extra Virgin Olive Oil

Breakfast Bowl
- Mixed Greens
- A handful of Parsley minced
- A handful of Cilantro minced
- Avocado

Directions:
Chickpea Scramble
1. Pour chickpeas and a little of the water they're in into a bowl. With a fork, mash chickpeas gently, leaving some whole. Mix in the turmeric, salt, and pepper until well mixed.
2. After that, mince the garlic and dice the onion. Using a sprinkle of olive oil, heat a pan over medium heat. To begin, sauté the onions until tender. Then add the garlic and sauté for approximately a minute, or until the garlic is fragrant. Take care not to brown the garlic!
3. When the onions and garlic are soft, add the mashed chickpeas and cook for about 5 minutes.

Breakfast Bowls
1. Make the breakfast bowls. Top the chickpea scramble with some mixed greens in the bottom of the bowls. Garnish with cilantro and parsley, if desired. Serve with pieces of avocado.
2. Enjoy!

Nutrition Facts: Calories: 172 | Carbohydrates: 17 g | Protein: 37 g | Fat: 49 g | Cholesterol: 90 mg

243. 3-INGREDIENT CHOCOLATE CEREAL

Prep Time: 30 minutes
Cook Time: 30 minutes
Total Time: 60 minutes
Servings: 4

Ingredients:
- 2 cups rolled oats, blended into flour
- 1/4 cup cocoa powder
- 1 cup date paste – 15 Medjool dates blended with 1 cup hot water

Directions:
1. Preheat the oven to 350°F.
2. In a large mixing basin, add the oat flour, cocoa powder, and date paste and whisk until a thick dough forms.
3. Pinch out approximately a teaspoon of the dough and form it into a tiny sphere; place on a prepared baking sheet and bake for 30 minutes.
4. Allow the cereal to rest on the counter for at least 2 hours before serving - this is when it becomes crispy.
5. Store at room temperature in a Tupperware container. It will soften when kept, so you may need to toast it short again after storage if you want it to be very crisp.

Nutrition Facts: Calories: 97 | Carbohydrates: 1 g | Protein: 7 g | Fat: 2 g | Cholesterol: 168 mg

244. VEGGIE QUICHE WITH SWEET POTATO CRUST

Prep Time: 10 minutes
Cook Time: 50 minutes
Total Time: 60 minutes
Servings: 3

Ingredients:
- 2 medium sweet potatoes
- 2 tablespoon olive oil
- 2 small yellow onion (finely chopped)
- 3 minced garlic cloves
- 3 cup cherry tomatoes (halved)
- 3 cups spinach
- 12 oz firm silken tofu
- 2 Tablespoon nutritional yeast
- 2 Tablespoon olive oil
- 2 garlic clove
- ¼ tablespoon sea salt
- ¼ tablespoon
- ¼ tablespoon ground sage
- Chopped green onion for garnish (optional)

Directions:
1. Preheat the oven to 375°F. Nonstick cooking sprays the bottom of a 9-inch (standard) pie plate.
2. Sweet potatoes should be peeled and cut into 18-inch rounds. Form a "crust" in your dish by layering the rounds (see photo). To make the upper layer, cut rounds in half. Spray the sweet potatoes well with nonstick cooking spray (I used this one) and season generously with sea salt and pepper.
3. 20 minutes in the oven
4. Begin preparing your vegetables while the sweet potato crust bakes. Heat the oil in a medium pan over medium/high heat and add the onions. After a minute, add the garlic and split tomatoes and sauté for another minute. Cook for another 2 minutes. Cook until the spinach is completely wilted. Remove the pan from the heat and set it aside.

5. To prepare the tofu filling, combine the tofu, nutritional yeast, olive oil, garlic, s&p, and ground sage in a food processor or blender. Blend until the mixture is totally smooth.
6. Mix in the tofu filling until it is well mixed with the vegetables.
7. When the potato crust is done, add your filling and level the top.
8. Bake for 30 minutes, or until the filling begins to color.
9. Allow cooling for 5 minutes after removing from the oven.
10. Cut into slices and serve. Enjoy!

Nutrition Facts: Calories: 212 | Carbohydrates: 15 g | Protein: 17 g | Fat: 1 g | Cholesterol: 83 mg

245. BLUEBERRY ALMOND OATMEAL

Prep Time: 5 minutes
Cook Time: 10 minutes
Total Time: 15 minutes
Servings: 2

Ingredients:
- 2 cup oats
- 2 cup oat milk
- 2 cups of water
- 1/2 cup frozen blueberries
- Toppings
- 2 tablespoon blueberries
- 3 tablespoon almonds chopped
- 3 tablespoon lemon juice
- 3 tablespoon maple syrup

Directions:
1. Cook the oats with the oat milk, water, and frozen blueberries over medium heat until the desired (thick) consistency is reached. It usually takes about ten minutes.
2. Add lemon juice, maple syrup, fresh blueberries, and sliced almonds over the top.

Nutrition Facts: Calories: 238 | Carbohydrates: 10 g | Protein: 14 g | Fat: 16 g | Cholesterol: 28 mg

246. GRANOLA YOGURT BREAKFAST TRIFLE

Prep Time: 5 minutes
Cook Time: 5 minutes
Total Time: 10 minutes
Servings: 2

Ingredients:
- 8 tablespoons of vegan yogurt
- 6 tablespoons of granola
- 2 tablespoons of nut mix
- 2 tablespoons of berries

Directions:
1. In a glass, layer your favorite granola.
2. Mix in the yogurt.
3. Enjoy!

Nutrition Facts: Calories: 1244 | Carbohydrates: 24 g | Protein: 64 g | Fat: 103 g | Cholesterol: 62 mg

247. LIME MINT SMOOTHIE

Prep Time: 5 minutes
Cook Time: 5 minutes
Total Time: 10 minutes
Servings: 2

Ingredients:
- 2,5 medium ripe bananas
- 2 cup oat milk
- 2 whole lime
- lime's juice
- 8 mint leaves
- 2 tablespoon maple syrup
- 6 ice cubes

Directions:
1. Put all ingredients in a blender.
2. Blend until smooth. (1-2 minutes)

Nutrition Facts: Calories: 485 | Carbohydrates: 2 g | Protein: 29 g | Fat: 38 g | Cholesterol: 19 mg

CHAPTER 13: LUNCH (FIBER-RICH)

248. BLACK BEANS AND AVOCADO TOASTS

Prep Time: 5 minutes
Cook Time: 15 minutes
Total Time: 20 minutes
Servings: 2

Ingredients:
- 2 slices of bread of your choice
- ½ avocado
- 4 tablespoons boiled black beans
- 2 tablespoon chopped green onions
- ½ lime
- ¼ teaspoon sea salt

Directions:
1. Mash the avocado and spread it on the bread pieces.
2. Serve with black beans and green onion on top.
3. Sprinkle salt and lemon juice on top of each.
4. Serve as fast as possible!

Nutrition Facts: Calories: 64 | Carbohydrates: 0 g | Protein: 5 g | Fat: 17 g | Cholesterol: 20 mg

249. APPLES N' OATS BREAKFAST SMOOTHIE

Prep Time: 10 minutes
Cook Time: 10 minutes
Total Time: 20 minutes
Servings: 4

Ingredients:
- 2 cup milk of choice (non-dairy or dairy)
- 2 large or 2 small apples, any variety
- 1/3 cup old fashioned rolled oats
- 2 Tablespoons hemp hearts (can substitute chia or flax s)
- 3 Tablespoon almond butter
- 1/2 teaspoon ground cinnamon
- 1/2 cup ice (optional, to make it cold)

Directions:
1. In a blender, combine the milk and oats. Allow the oats to soften for a few minutes.
2. Peel and core the apple. If desired, peel.
3. Fill the blender halfway with the remaining ingredients. Puree until completely smooth. Can be made a day ahead of time and refrigerated, covered.

Note: If adding flax or chia seeds, add 1/4 to 1/2 cup extra liquid to prevent the smoothie from becoming too thick.

Nutrition Facts: Calories: 358 | Carbohydrates: 3 g | Protein: 33 g | Fat: 12 g | Cholesterol: 81 mg

250. PACKED BURRITO

Prep Time: 10 minutes
Cook Time: 10 minutes
Total Time: 20 minutes
Servings: 4

Ingredients:
- ½ of medium red onion (chopped)
- Two garlic cloves (minced)
- 12 oz of extra firm tofu (pressed, see notes)
- 2 Tablespoon olive oil
- ¼ tablespoon turmeric
- ¼ tablespoon cumin
- Sea salt & to taste
- ½ cup of black beans
- ½ of avocado (chopped into small pieces)
- ⅓ cup of salsa any of choice (I used pico de gallo)
- Three large whole wheat tortillas

Directions:
1. Heat the oil in a medium-sized pan over medium heat. Once cooked, add your onions and season with salt and pepper. Cook until the mixture has been cooked down and color gently (about 4-5 minutes). Cook for another minute, frequently stirring, after adding your garlic.

2. Tofu should be added at this point (crumble it with your hands, see picture). Stir in the turmeric, cumin, and another sprinkle of sea salt. Stir until completely mixed. Turn off the heat.
3. To construct your burritos, arrange all of your ingredients (allowing room on both sides, as seen in the photo) and roll up! Enjoy!
4. You may freeze them by placing them in a tight plastic bag.

Nutrition Facts: Calories: 519 | Carbohydrates: 17 g | Protein: 27 g | Fat: 18 g | Cholesterol: 251 mg

251. <u>BLOOD ORANGE CHIA PUDDING</u>

Prep Time: 5 minutes
Cook Time: 5 minutes
Total Time: 10 minutes
Servings: 2

Ingredients:
- 3 blood oranges, peeled (400 grams)
- 3/4 cup lite coconut milk
- 1/2 teaspoon cinnamon
- 1/3 cup chia s

Directions:
1. In a Vita mix, high-powered blender, or food processor, combine the oranges, coconut milk, and cinnamon. About 1 minute, process until smooth and all ingredients are mixed.
2. Transfer to a resealable medium-sized bowl. Stir in the chia seeds until well blended. Cover and place in the refrigerator for 3 hours or overnight.
3. Serve plain or with preferred toppings.
4. Enjoy!

Nutrition Facts: Calories: 127 | Carbohydrates: 14 g | Protein: 8 g | Fat: 12 g | Cholesterol: 162 mg

252. <u>BLUEBERRY COCONUT SMOOTHIE BOWL</u>

Prep Time: 5 minutes
Cook Time: 5 minutes
Total Time: 10 minutes
Servings: 1

Ingredients:
- 3 tablespoon (15 g) unsweetened shredded coconut
- 3/4 cup unsweetened almond milk
- serving vegan vanilla protein powder
- 2 cup (125 g) frozen zucchini chunks
- 1/2 cup (50 g) frozen cauliflower
- 1/2 cup (75 g) frozen blueberries
- tablespoon Ceylon cinnamon (optional)
- pinch of Himalayan crystal salt or another unrefined sea salt (optional, do not use table salt)

Directions:
1. In a high-speed blender, combine the coconut and liquid and mix for about a minute on high.
2. Add the other ingredients and process until thick and creamy. To keep it from thinning out, don't over-mix or leave it in the blender for too long, since the heat from the blender can melt it.
3. Scoop the mixture into a bowl, top with your preferred toppings, and serve with a spoon!

Nutrition Facts: Calories: 206 | Carbohydrates: 36 g | Protein: 21 g | Fat: 19 g | Cholesterol: 26 mg

253. <u>NO-BAKE APRICOT OAT PROTEIN BARS</u>

Prep Time: 30 minutes
Cook Time: 30 minutes
Total Time: 60 minutes
Servings: 10

Ingredients:
- 1/2 cup pumpkin s

- 4 cup gluten free rolled oats
- 1/2 cup flax
- 3 cup dried Turkish Apricots (+ extra chopped for topping)
- pinch of sea salt
- hot water
- 1/2 tablespoon cinnamon
- 1/4 cup of maple syrup (or honey if not vegan)
- 1/2 cup of vanilla protein powder (vegan)
- optional toppings – 1/4 cup Optional melting Dark Chocolate (vegan/gluten free)

Directions:
1. Combine the pumpkin, gluten-free oats, and flax. Blend until a "mealy" batter is produced (in a blender or food processor).
2. Pour the batter into a mixing basin.
3. Next, blend/pulse the apricots until they are finely chopped/diced. Blend in with the oats. Combine the protein powder, salt, and cinnamon in a mixing bowl.
4. Combine your maple syrup or honey, 1/3 cup boiling water, and vanilla essence in a separate small mixing dish. Stir everything together and add it to the dry ingredients (the apricot/oat/protein mixture).
5. Mix well with your hands, then press into a baking dish. Top with additional chopped apricots and oats. Add vegan chocolate (dark chocolate) here if desired. Simply microwave vegan chocolate chips for 45 seconds, mix, and sprinkle over bars.
6. Allow bars to chill in the refrigerator to set—approximately 30 minutes. Notes about batter texture can be found here.
7. When the batter has been set, cut it into 10 squares.
8. Store in the refrigerator.

Nutrition Facts: Calories: 232 | Carbohydrates: 25 g | Protein: 13 g | Fat: 1.7 g | Cholesterol: 23 mg

254. **SPRINGTIME TOFU SCRAMBLE**

Prep Time: 15 minutes
Cook Time: 17 minutes
Total Time: 32 minutes
Servings: 4

Ingredients:
- 2 tablespoon olive oil or virgin coconut oil
- 3 clove garlic, minced
- 3 leek thoroughly washed, halved, and thinly sliced (white and light green parts only)
- 2 cups baby spinach
- 4 small yellow squash quartered and sliced (about 1 ½ cups)
- 6 oz baby Bella mushrooms washed, destemmed, and sliced
- 14 oz firm sprouted tofu
- ½ teaspoons turmeric
- tablespoon nutritional yeast
- ½ teaspoon truffle salt or Kala namak (i.e., black salt)
- ¼ teaspoon sea salt
- tablespoons fresh chives

Directions:
1. Heat the oil in a large skillet over medium-low heat. Add the garlic, leek, spinach, squash, and mushrooms after that. Cook, occasionally stirring, for 10-12 minutes, or until the vegetables are soft.
2. Crumble the tofu and add the turmeric, nutritional yeast, truffle salt, salt, and black pepper to the pan. Cook for an additional 5 minutes.
3. Remove from the heat and toss in the chives.
4. If preferred, serve with avocado toast.

Nutrition Facts: Calories: 182 | Carbohydrates: 11 g | Protein: 10 g | Fat: 72 g | Cholesterol: 182 mg

255. **DATE-SWEETENED BANANA BREAD**

Prep Time: 20 minutes
Cook Time: 50 minutes
Total Time: 70 minutes
Servings: 8

Ingredients:
- Two flax eggs (2 tablespoons flax meal + 6 tablespoons water)*
- 2 cups gluten-free oat flour
- 2 teaspoon cinnamon
- 2 teaspoon baking powder
- 1/2 teaspoon baking soda
- ½ teaspoon salt
- 1 large ripe & spotty bananas, mashed (about 1 1/2 cups)
- + 1 banana to top, sliced it in half lengthwise (optional)
- cup pitted Medjool dates, packed
- ½ cup unsweetened non-dairy milk
- 1 ½ –2 teaspoons of pure vanilla extract (I used 2)
- One teaspoon of apple cider vinegar

Directions:
1. Preheat the oven to 350°F and line or lightly grease a 9-inch bread pan with parchment paper. Stir together the flax meal and the water. Set aside for about 15 minutes to thicken.
2. Combine the oat flour, baking soda, baking powder, salt, cinnamon, and if using in a large mixing basin. Set aside after thoroughly mixing.
3. Combine the dates, almond milk, vanilla essence, and apple cider vinegar in a food processor. Process until smooth, then use a spoon to incorporate the mashed banana and flax egg. Stir the date and banana mixture into the dry ingredients until a batter forms.
4. Pour the batter into the prepared loaf pan and top with the optional banana, sliced side up, if preferred (refer to photos in post).
5. Bake for 50-60 minutes, or until a toothpick inserted into the center comes out clean. Remove from the oven and set aside to cool fully before slicing.

Nutrition Facts: Calories: 429 | Carbohydrates: 19 g | Protein: 13 g | Fat: 27 g | Cholesterol: 10 mg

256. <u>2 MINUTE FLOURLESS ENGLISH MUFFIN</u>

Prep Time: 1 minute
Cook Time: 2 minutes
Total Time: 3 minutes
Servings: 1

Ingredients:
- 1/3 cup rolled oats gluten free, if necessary- For PALEO/GRAIN FREE option, see link above
- 2 tablespoon chia
- ½ teaspoon baking powder
- 2 tablespoon unsweetened applesauce
- 3 tablespoon milk of choice
- Optional: a pinch of salt

Directions:
7. Combine the oats, chia seeds, baking powder, and salt in a blender. Blend on high until the mixture is finely ground.
8. Transfer to a mixing dish and stir in the applesauce and non-dairy milk to make a sticky dough.
9. Place the dough in a ramekin and press it down.
10. Microwave on high for 2 minutes.
11. Allow it to cool for 5 minutes before taking it from the ramekin.
12. Cut in half, toast, and serve with desired toppings.

Nutrition Facts: Calories: 174 | Carbohydrates: 22 g | Protein: 7 g | Fat: 6 g | Cholesterol: 19 mg

257. <u>BLUEBERRY CHIA JAM</u>

Prep Time: 20 minutes
Cook Time: 20 minutes
Total Time: 40 minutes
Servings: 4

Ingredients:
- 3 cups fresh blueberry
- 3-4 tablespoons maple syrup
- 2 tablespoons chia s
- ½ teaspoon vanilla extract (optional)

Directions:
1. In a medium nonstick saucepan over medium heat, combine blueberries and 3 tablespoons maple syrup and bring to a low boil. Reduce the heat slightly and continue to cook for approximately 5 minutes, stirring often, or until all of the berries have darkened and become glossy, like small marbles. Mash the berries with a potato masher, keeping some whole for texture.
2. Reduce the heat to low and stir in the chia seeds. Allow it to boil for about 15 minutes, stirring regularly, or until thickened—it will thicken further in the fridge.
3. Take the pan off the heat and whisk in the vanilla extract.

Nutrition Facts: Calories: 134 | Carbohydrates: 29 g | Protein: 2 g | Fat: 2 g | Cholesterol: 61 mg

258. PEANUT BUTTER CHIA OVERNIGHT OATS

Prep Time: 10 minutes
Cook Time: 30 minutes
Total Time: 40 minutes
Servings: 1

Ingredients:
Scale
- 3/4 cup rolled oats
- 2 tablespoons chia s
- 1/2 teaspoon cinnamon
- pinch of sea salt
- Twp cup of unsweetened vanilla almond milk (or any plant milk)*
- 1/2 cup filtered water
- 3 teaspoon vanilla extract (optional)
- 2 ripe bananas, mashed (but leave a few banana coins for topping!)
- Three tablespoons of PB Fit powder + 1 ½ tablespoons of water (or any nut butter, to taste)
- 1–2 tablespoons maple syrup or agave for extra sweetness

Extras/Toppings
- crushed almonds
- sliced banana coins
- extra sprinkles of cinnamon!
- cacao nibs (optional)
- coconut flakes

Directions:
1. In a mason jar, combine the oats, chia seeds, cinnamon, and sea salt. Mix in the almond milk, water, vanilla extract, and mashed banana. Stir everything together until it's smooth.
2. In a small mixing dish, combine the PB powder and water until smooth. You may double the ingredients to get even more peanut butter taste! Pour the "peanut butter" mixture into the mason jar. Toppings can be added now or in the morning!
3. Refrigerate for at least four hours or overnight. Using a spoon, dig in and enjoy!

Nutrition Facts: Calories: 55 | Carbohydrates: 10 g | Protein: 13 g | Fat: 1 g | Cholesterol: 10 mg

259. PUMPKIN PIE CHIA PUDDING

Prep Time: 10 minutes
Cook Time: 180 minutes
Total Time: 190 minutes
Servings: 2

Ingredients:
- 1/2 cup raw pecans
- 1/2 cups of pumpkin puree (canned or fresh)
- 1/2 cups almond milk
- 2 teaspoon cinnamon
- 1/2 teaspoon ground ginger
- 1/2 teaspoon nutmeg
- pinch of sea salt
- 1/4 cup chia s
- optional toppings: fresh fruit, nut butter, whipped cream, cinnamon

Directions:
1. Toasted pecans Allow a small skillet to heat up over medium-low heat for about 30 seconds. Toast the nuts for 4-5 minutes, stirring continuously, until golden brown.
2. In a high-powered blender or food processor, combine pecans, pumpkin, almond milk, cinnamon, ginger, nutmeg, and salt. About 1-2 minutes, process until smooth and all ingredients are mixed.
3. Transfer to a resealable medium-sized bowl. Stir in the chia seeds until well combined. Cover and place in the refrigerator for 3 hours or overnight.
4. Serve plain or with preferred toppings. Enjoy!

Nutrition Facts: Calories: 410 | Carbohydrates: 27 g | Protein: 38 g | Fat: 18 g | Cholesterol: 109 mg

260. <u>PUMPKIN PIE BUTTER</u>

Prep Time: 10 minutes
Cook Time: 50 minutes
Total Time: 60 minutes
Servings: 2

Ingredients:
- 2 1/2 cups packed freshly roasted pumpkin (see below for instructions - can also use canned if you like)
- 1/2 teaspoons cinnamon
- 1/2 teaspoon ginger
- 1/2 teaspoon nutmeg
- 1/2 teaspoon ground cloves
- 1/4 teaspoon salt
- 2 tablespoon maple syrup (optional - leave out for Whole30)

Directions:
1. If using fresh pumpkin, chop it into big pieces (skin on) and remove the seeds (keep them roasting!). Rub the flesh with a small amount of neutral oil (I use coconut oil) and roast for 45 minutes to an hour at 375 degrees Fahrenheit or until soft.
2. Toast when the pumpkin is almost done. Melt the butter in a medium pan over medium-low heat. And toast them for 3-6 minutes, stirring regularly, until they begin to brown and become aromatic. Remove from the heat and put aside.
3. Allow the pumpkin to cool for a few minutes before removing the meat from the skin. Then, in a high-powered blender, combine 2 1/2 cups of the flesh (squeeze it into a measuring cup to make sure you pack it in) (I used my Vitamix). Spices, maple syrup (optional), and salt Blend for 1–3 minutes, or until smooth and creamy. If desired, add extra spices or sugar. Refrigerate in a securely sealed glass jar for 2-3 weeks before serving.

Note: Pumpkin butter may be kept in the fridge for 2-3 weeks in a firmly sealed glass jar. It is also possible to freeze it for up to 6 months. For ease of usage, I recommend freezing in serving quantities of 2-3.

I adore using fresh pumpkins since the freshly roasted flavor is fantastic, and they are only available for a few months of the year. I recommend choosing sugar or pie pumpkins since they have the greatest flavor and natural sweetness. You'll need a good-sized pumpkin. Avoid using "jack-o-lantern" pumpkins. If you want, you may use canned pumpkin, but it will be less thick.

Nutrition Facts: Calories: 76 | Carbohydrates: 27 g | Protein: 11 g | Fat: 28 g | Cholesterol: 36 mg

261. <u>SPICED PUMPKIN GRANOLA</u>

Prep Time: 5 minutes
Cook Time: 25 minutes
Total Time: 30 minutes
Servings: 4

Ingredients:
- 2 cup raw pumpkin s
- 2/3 cup raw sunflower s
- 4 Tablespoons flax s
- 1/2 teaspoon cinnamon

- 4 teaspoon pumpkin spice (or homemade version below)
- 1/4 teaspoon sea salt or coarse kosher salt
- 1/4 cup maple syrup
- 1/3 to 1/2 cup unsweetened coconut

Directions:
1. Preheat the oven to 325 degrees F.
2. Set aside a baking sheet lined with parchment paper.
3. In a mixing bowl, combine all ingredients (except the coconut) in the order given. To mix, stir everything together.
4. Spread the mixture evenly on a baking sheet lined with parchment paper and bake for 20 minutes.
5. Bake for 20 minutes at 325 degrees Fahrenheit. (See also the notes)
6. Add the coconut to the pan and stir it in evenly with a spoon. Return the baking pan to the oven for an additional 5-7 minutes to roast the coconut.
7. Then, take the pan out of the oven and let the granola cool on the pan.
8. The granola should be ready to break into smaller pieces once it has cooled in the pan.
9. Enjoy with any optional mix-ins of your choice!

Nutrition Facts: Calories: 273 | Carbohydrates: 15 g | Protein: 7 g | Fat: 1 g | Cholesterol: 28 mg

262. <u>COCONUT ALMOND PROTEIN BARS</u>

Prep Time: 15 minutes
Cook Time: 15 minutes
Total Time: 30 minutes
Servings: 8

Ingredients:
- 2-1/2 cups of raw almonds
- 1/2 cup of unsweetened coconut flakes
- 1/4 cup of dried mango (about 4-5 pieces). It should be noted that dried apricots and pineapple may be used instead.
- 1/4 cup or 2 scoops of (60 grams) protein powder of choice
- Three teaspoons of cinnamon (optional)
- Pinch of sea salt
- 1/3 to 1/2 cup honey or maple syrup
- 1/3 to 1/2 cup hot water (purified)
- Four teaspoons pure vanilla extract

Directions:
1. To begin, place the almonds and coconut in a high-powered blender or food processor and pulse until an almond meal-like texture is created.
2. Set aside in a large mixing basin.
3. The dried mango is then ground up. They might be difficult to digest at times. If you don't have a high-powered blender or food processor, chop the mango into smaller pieces using a sharp knife.
4. Remove the dried mango from the food processor and combine it with the almond coconut mixture. Combine the protein powder, cinnamon, and salt in a mixing bowl. Set aside.
5. Separately, in a small mixing dish. Combine honey or maple syrup, boiling water, and vanilla extract in a mixing bowl. Stir to mix before adding to the dry ingredients.
6. If the batter is overly thick, simply add additional boiling water or honey. If it's too moist, add additional protein powder or your preferred flour. Mix thoroughly with your hands, then press into an 8x8 baking dish lined with parchment paper. Allow bars to chill in the fridge for 1 hour or more before cutting into squares.
7. Refrigerate after opening and eat within 5 to 7 days.

Nutrition Facts: Calories: 273 | Carbohydrates: 20 g | Protein: 19 g | Fat: 12 g | Cholesterol: 37 mg

263. <u>GRAIN-FREE GRANOLA CLUSTERS</u>

Prep Time: 10 minutes
Cook Time: 25 minutes

Total Time: 35 minutes
Servings: 8

Ingredients:
- 2 cup slivered almonds
- 1/3 cup semi sweet or dark chocolate chips (vegan) or sugar free chocolate chips.
- optional 1–2 tablespoons of chia or flax
- optional 1 teaspoon vanilla extract
- 1/4 teaspoon kosher salt
- 1/4 teaspoon cinnamon
- 1/4 cup pure maple syrup or raw honey

Directions:
1. Preheat the oven to 325°F.
2. Set aside a baking sheet lined with parchment paper.
3. In a mixing dish, combine all of the ingredients in the order given. To mix, stir everything together.
4. Spread the mixture evenly onto the prepared baking sheet and bake for 20 minutes.
5. Bake for 25-30 minutes at 325°F. My time was 28 minutes. When they are golden and the chocolate is somewhat melted, you'll know it's done.
6. Then, take the pan out of the oven and let the granola cool on the pan. Do not make any contact! The chocolate and maple syrup should have melted together, tying everything together.
7. The granola should be ready to break into big pieces once it has cooled in the pan. Granola clusters are another name for granola clusters.
8. Keep in an airtight jar for up to two weeks.

Nutrition Facts: Calories: 168 | Carbohydrates: 13 g | Protein: 3 g | Fat: 12 g | Cholesterol: 0.3 mg

264. **TOASTED COCONUT AND BERRY GRAIN**

Prep Time: 10 minutes
Cook Time: 35 minutes
Total Time: 45 minutes

Servings: 6

Ingredients:
- 1 cup larger size whole mixed (like brazil, hazelnut, or)
- 1 cup raw almonds
- 1/2 cup pumpkin s
- 1/4 cup coconut oil
- 1/4 to 1/3 cup maple syrup
- 2 tablespoon vanilla
- 2 tablespoon cinnamon
- 1/2 tablespoon ground ginger
- dash of sea salt
- 2/3 cup unsweetened coconut flakes
- 1 ½ cup to 1 ¼ cup dried berries (blueberry, cranberry, etc.)
- Optional chia s (2 tablespoons)

Directions:
1. Preheat the oven to 325°F. Preheat the oven to 350°F. Line a baking sheet with parchment paper.
2. Combine your /almonds in a blender or food processor. Pulse approximately 5-8 times until the ingredients are chopped but not ground.
3. Transfer to a large mixing dish and stir in your pumpkins.
4. Combine the coconut oil, extract, and maple syrup in a separate basin. Pour this over the and toss to combine. Then add your spices and stir until evenly covered.
5. Spread the nut mixture equally on the baking sheet and top with a pinch of sea salt. Maybe a quarter teaspoon?
6. Bake for 15 minutes in a preheated oven.
7. Remove from the oven and toss the /s on the tray to turn the sides. Return to the oven for another fifteen minutes of baking.
8. Remove from oven, stir /s, and then put in your coconut. You may place the coconut on the same baking pan as the nuts and syrup or a different baking dish. Just make sure it's evenly distributed on the tray.
9. Continue baking for another five-eight minute, or until the coconut is golden brown.
10. Remove and set aside to cool.

11. After cooling, add the coconut/nut granola to a mixing bowl and stir it around a bit more. Mix in the dried berries and toss everything together.
12. Finish with any more spices and optional chia.
13. Keep in an airtight container or gift jars.

Nutrition Facts: Calories: 200 | Carbohydrates: 8 g | Protein: 4 g | Fat: 13 g | Cholesterol: 263 mg

265. BERRY SOFT SERVE & VANILLA CHIA PUDDING PARFAIT

Prep Time: 15 minutes
Cook Time: 630 minutes
Total Time: 40 minutes
Servings: 2

Ingredients:
Vanilla Chia Pudding
- ¼ cups unsweetened plant milk
- ¼ cup plus 1 tablespoon chia s
- ½ to 2 tablespoons pure maple syrup
- 2 teaspoon pure vanilla extract
- Berry Soft Serve
- 3 cups frozen strawberries
- ½ cup frozen blueberries
- to 2 Medjool dates, pitted (optional to sweeten)

Topping Ideas
- coconut flakes
- sliced strawberries
- blueberries

Directions:
Vanilla Chia Pudding
1. In an airtight jar or container, vigorously mix the plant milk, chia seeds, maple syrup, and vanilla until the chia seeds are evenly dispersed throughout the liquid. To thicken, place in the refrigerator for at least 8 hours or overnight.
2. In the morning, mix the chia pudding thoroughly. If it's too thin, add 1 tablespoon of chia seeds at a time to thicken. If it's too thick, thin with additional plant milk, 1 tablespoon at a time.
3. Soft Serve Berry
4. Just before serving, make the soft serve. Combine the frozen strawberries, sugar, and lemon juice in a food processor. Blueberries, dates (if using) and process until smooth and sorbet-like, stopping to scrape down the sides as required. To start things rolling, you may need to add a very small amount of plant milk. To retain a thick, soft-serve texture, add 1 spoonful at a time and as little as possible.

Assemble
1. Layer the chia pudding and soft berry serve in two jars or parfait glasses, one after the other. Serve immediately after sprinkling with preferred toppings.

Nutrition Facts: Calories: 396 | Carbohydrates: 10 g | Protein: 20 g | Fat: 10 g | Cholesterol: 81 mg

266. RAW GRANOLA CLUSTERS, COCONUT WHIPPED CREAM, AND DREAMY BERRY PARFAIT

Prep Time: 25 minutes
Cook Time: 5 minutes
Total Time: 30 minutes
Servings: 4

Ingredients:
For the Raw Cinnamon Almond Crumble
- ½ cup raw almonds
- ½ cup pitted Medjool dates
- ½ cup gluten-free rolled oats
- ½ teaspoon cinnamon
- ⅛ teaspoon cardamom
- 2 teaspoon vanilla extract

For the Coconut Whipped Cream
- 3 cups of coconut cream

- 2 tablespoons of powdered sugar (or stevia, to taste)
- one vanilla bean

Additional Ingredients:
- ½ cup 5-minute vegan caramel sauce
- 2 cup quartered and pitted sweet cherries
- 2 cup raspberries
- 3 cup blueberries
- ½ cup quartered strawberries

Directions:

To Make the Raw Cinnamon Almond Crumble
1. Combine the almonds, dates, oats, cinnamon, cardamom, and vanilla essence in a mixing bowl. Process for 1-2 minutes, or until a crumbly, somewhat sticky substance develops, after pulsing 10 times. Refrigerate until ready to use, covered.

To Make the Coconut Whipped Cream
1. Combine the coconut cream, powdered sugar or stevia, and vanilla beans in a medium mixing bowl. Whip the coconut cream for 3-4 minutes on high speed. Or until a thick whipped cream develops, using a hand mixer with whisk attachments. Refrigerate until ready to use, covered.

To Assemble
1. Layer the berries in small bowls or jars, then top with the crumble, a dollop of coconut whipped cream, and a drizzle of the caramel sauce. Repeat once more, then top with fresh berries.
2. Serve right away.
3. Keep any leftovers in the refrigerator.

Nutrition Facts: Calories: 133 | Carbohydrates: 19 g | Protein: 22 g | Fat: 18 g | Cholesterol: 30 mg

267. **CREAMY RASPBERRY, COCONUT & CHIA SHAKE**

Prep Time: 10 minutes
Cook Time: 10 minutes
Total Time: 20 minutes
Servings: 2

Ingredients:

- ½ cups frozen raspberries
- ⅓ cup full-fat canned coconut milk, chilled
- cup unsweetened oat milk or almond milk
- ½ cup ice
- 4 soft Medjool dates, pitted
- 3 tablespoon chia
- 2 teaspoon pure vanilla extract

Directions:
1. Combine all of the ingredients in a high-powered blender and blend until smooth.

Nutrition Facts: Calories: 276 | Carbohydrates: 9 g | Protein: 38 g | Fat: 10 g | Cholesterol: 28 mg

268. **RAW CHERRY-APPLE PIE**

Prep Time: 25 minutes
Cook Time: 25 minutes
Total Time: 50 minutes
Servings: 2

Ingredients:

- 3 cups fresh or thawed frozen sweet cherries, pitted and divided
- 1 large crisp apple, cored, peeled, and diced
- 4 dates, pitted
- 2 tablespoons chia s

Topping Ideas
- raw almonds
- dried mulberries
- hemp s
- cacao nibs

Directions:
1. 1 cup of the cherries, diced, should be placed in a medium airtight container with the diced apple.
2. Combine the remaining 2 cups of sweet cherries and the dates in a high-speed blender. Process or mix for 1 to 2 minutes, or until smooth, occasionally stopping to scrape down the sides. Pour the cherry sauce into the container with the chopped cherries and apple, then mix the chia seeds.
3. Refrigerate for at least an hour, if not more, before serving.

4. Divide the apple mixture into two bowls and top with raw raisins, cranberries, and hemp seeds.
5. Serve immediately and enjoy.
6. Keep any leftovers in the refrigerator.

Nutrition Facts: Calories: 190 | Carbohydrates: 22 g | Protein: 12 g | Fat: 33 g | Cholesterol: 16 mg

269. STRAWBERRY-WATERMELON REFRESHER JUICE

Prep Time: 125 minutes
Cook Time: 20 minutes
Total Time: 40 minutes
Servings: 1

Ingredients:
- 3 cups fresh watermelon, cubed
- ½ cups fresh strawberries, hulled
- 2 small handfuls of fresh mint leaves

Directions:
1. For 2-3 hours, place the watermelon cubes in the freezer. They should be icy but not entirely frozen.
2. In a blender, combine the frosted watermelon, fresh strawberries, and mint leaves. Blend for 1-2 minutes, or until the mixture is smooth and foamy.
3. Fill a large glass with ice and enjoy!

Nutrition Facts: Calories: 55 | Carbohydrates: 10 g | Protein: 13 g | Fat: 1 g | Cholesterol: 10 mg

270. BLUEBERRY BIRCHER POTS

Prep Time: 10 minutes
Cook Time: 25 minutes
Total Time: 35 minutes
Servings: 1

Ingredients:
- small apple
- tablespoon whole oats
- tablespoon low-fat natural yogurt
- some blueberries

Directions:
1. 1 small apple, grated, 2 tablespoon whole oats, 2 tablespoons low-fat natural yogurt In a pot, layer with blueberries.

Nutrition Facts: Calories: 222 | Carbohydrates: 38 g | Protein: 13 g | Fat: 20 g | Cholesterol: 8 mg

271. JACKET POTATOES WITH HOME-BAKED BEANS

Prep Time: 10 minutes
Cook Time: 90 minutes
Total Time: 100 minutes
Servings: 4

Ingredients:
- 4 baking potatoes
- 2 tablespoon sunflower oil
- 1 carrot, diced
- 1 celery stalk, diced
- 400g can haricot beans, drained
- 2 tomatoes, chopped
- 2 tablespoon paprika - choose sweet or hot depending on taste
- 2 tablespoon Worcestershire sauce
- 3 tablespoon chopped chives, to serve

Directions:

1. Preheat the oven to 200°C/180°C fan/gas 6. Scrub and dry the potatoes thoroughly before pricking them numerous times with a fork. Bake for 1-12 hours, or until they feel soft when pressed, straight on the oven shelf.
2. After 30 minutes, heat the oil in a skillet and sauté the carrot and celery for 10 minutes, or until softened. Cook for another 5 minutes, or until the beans, tomatoes, and paprika are softened and pulpy. Cook for 5 minutes more after adding 100ml water and the Worcestershire sauce, cover and keep heated.
3. Split the potatoes open and spoon in the beans. Serve garnished with chives.

Nutrition Facts: Calories: 237 | Carbohydrates: 45 g | Protein: 19 g | Fat: 4 g | Cholesterol: 50 mg

272. **PEA & BROAD BEAN SHAKSHUKA**

Prep Time: 20 minutes
Cook Time: 30 minutes
Total Time: 50 minutes
Servings: 4

Ingredients:
- ½ bunch asparagus spears
- 200g sprouting broccoli
- 2 tablespoon olive oil
- spring onions, finely sliced
- 2 tablespoon cumin
- ripe tomatoes, chopped
- small pack parsley, finely chopped
- 50g shelled peas
- 50g podded broad beans
- 4 large eggs
- 50g pea shoots
- Greek yogurt and flatbreads, to serve

Directions:

1. Trim or break the asparagus's woody ends and thinly slice the spears, leaving the tips approximately 2cm at the top intact. Similarly, finely slice the broccoli, leaving the heads and roughly 2cm of stem intact. In a frying pan, heat the oil. Stir in the spring onions, sliced asparagus, and sliced broccoli until the vegetables soften slightly, add the cumin, cayenne pepper, tomatoes (with juices), parsley, and lots of salt. Cover and simmer for 5 minutes to form a base sauce, then add the asparagus spears, broccoli heads, peas, and broad beans, cover again, and cook for another 2 minutes.
2. Make four dips using the mixture. Break an egg into each dip, surround it with half the pea shoots, season generously, cover with a lid, and heat until the egg whites are barely set. Serve with the remaining pea shoots, a tablespoon of yogurt, several flatbreads, and top with another teaspoon of cayenne, if desired.

Nutrition Facts: Calories: 172 | Carbohydrates: 7 g | Protein: 13 g | Fat: 5 g | Cholesterol: 27 mg

273. **LENTIL FRITTERS**

Prep Time: 15 minutes
Cook Time: 10 minutes
Total Time: 25 minutes
Servings: 2

Ingredients:
- 300g leftover basic lentils
- a handful of chopped coriander
- 2 chopped spring onion
- 50g gram flour
- 2 carrots
- 2 courgettes
- 1 handful of coriander
- ½ tablespoon oil
- juice of 1 lime
- 3 tablespoon rape oil

Directions:

1. Set aside the remaining lentils with the chopped coriander, spring onion, and gram flour. Cut the carrots and courgettes into long ribbons with a peeler, then mix the coriander in oil and lime juice.
2. In a frying pan, heat the rape oil. Flatten four dollops of the lentil mixture into patties. Fry until golden on each side, then serve with the ribbon salad.

Nutrition Facts: Calories: 162 | Carbohydrates: 22 g | Protein: 18 g | Fat: 12 g | Cholesterol: 137 mg

2. Meanwhile, in a food processor (or a bowl with a stick blender), blitz the remaining beans and tomatoes, garlic, and basil until smooth, then mix in the Parmesan. Cook for 1 minute after stirring the sauce, then ladle half into bowls or pour into a flask for a packed lunch. The rest of the ingredients should be chilled. I will keep it for a few days.

Nutrition Facts: Calories: 162 | Carbohydrates: 15 g | Protein: 13 g | Fat: 10 g | Cholesterol: 36 mg

274. **SUMMER PISTOU**

Prep Time: 10 minutes
Cook Time: 25 minutes
Total Time: 35 minutes
Servings: 4

Ingredients:
- 4 tablespoon rape oil
- 2 leeks, finely sliced
- 2 large courgettes, finely diced
- 1l boiling vegetable stock (made from scratch or with reduced-salt bouillon)
- 400g can cannellini or haricot beans, drained
- 200g green beans, chopped
- 4 tomatoes, chopped
- 2 garlic cloves, finely chopped
- small pack basil
- 40g freshly grated parmesan

Directions:
1. In a big pan, heat the oil and cook the leeks and courgette for 5 minutes to soften. Pour in the stock, add three-quarters of the haricot beans and the green beans and half of the tomatoes, and cook for 5-8 minutes, or until the vegetables are soft.

275. **WINTER VEGETABLE & LENTIL SOUP**

Prep Time: 10 minutes
Cook Time: 30 minutes
Total Time: 40 minutes
Servings: 2

Ingredients:
- 85g dried red lentils
- 2 carrots, quartered lengthways then diced
- 3 sticks celery, sliced
- 2 small leeks, sliced
- 2 tablespoon tomato purée
- 2 tablespoon fresh thyme leaves
- 1 large garlic cloves, chopped
- 2 tablespoon vegetable bouillon powder
- 2 heaped tablespoon ground coriander

Directions:
1. Place all of the ingredients in a large pan. Pour in 1½ liters of hot water and stir thoroughly.
2. Cook for 30 minutes, or until the veggies and lentils are soft.
3. Ladle into bowls and serve immediately, or blitz a third of the soup with a hand blender or in a food processor if you like a thick texture.

Nutrition Facts: Calories: 152 | Carbohydrates: 38 g | Protein: 40 g | Fat: 53 g | Cholesterol: 20 mg

276. BAKED SWEET POTATOES & BEANS

Prep Time: 10 minutes
Cook Time: 25 minutes
Total Time: 35 minutes
Servings: 2

Ingredients:
- 4 small sweet potatoes
- 2 tablespoon smoked paprika, plus extra to serve
- 2 tablespoon olive oil
- 2 large onions, chopped
- 3 garlic cloves, crushed
- 2 tablespoon brown sugar
- 2 tablespoon red wine vinegar
- 1 splash of Worcestershire sauce (Lancashire sauce is a veggie option)
- x 400g cans mixed beans in water, drained
- 400g chopped tomatoes
- 1 tablespoon light soured cream, to serve

Directions:
1. Heat the oven to 200°C/180°C fan/gas 6 Pierce the sweet potatoes several times with a fork, then microwave on High for 8 minutes, or until tender. Rub with 1 tablespoon paprika, 1 tablespoon oil, and some spice. Place on a baking sheet and bake for 10-15 minutes, or until crispy.
2. In the meantime, prepare the beans. Cook until the onion is tender in the remaining oil. Cook for another 1-2 minutes, until sticky, with the garlic, sugar, vinegar, Worcestershire sauce, and remaining paprika. Cook until the sweet potatoes are tender, then add the beans, tomatoes, and a splash of water.
3. If desired, serve the sweet potatoes with the beans, a dollop of soured cream, and a sprinkle of paprika on top.

Nutrition Facts: Calories: 136 | Carbohydrates: 36 g | Protein: 29 g | Fat: 9 g | Cholesterol: 18 mg

DINNER (FIBER-RICH)

277. EASY PEA & SPINACH CARBONARA

Prep Time: 20 minutes
Cook Time: 30 minutes
Total Time: 50 minutes
Servings: 4

Ingredients:
- 1 ½ tablespoon extra-virgin olive oil
- ½ cup panko breadcrumbs, preferably whole-wheat
- 2 small clove garlic, minced
- 8 tablespoons grated Parmesan cheese, divided
- 2 tablespoons finely chopped fresh parsley
- 3 large egg yolks
- 3 large egg
- ¼ teaspoon salt
- (9 ounces) package fresh tagliatelle or linguine
- 8 cups baby spinach
- 2 cups of peas (fresh or frozen)

Directions:
1. In a large saucepan over high heat, bring 10 cups of water to a boil. Meanwhile, in a large pan over medium-high heat, heat the oil. Cook, often tossing, until the breadcrumbs and garlic are toasted, about 2 minutes. In a small bowl, combine 2 tablespoons of Parmesan and parsley. Set it aside.
2. Combine the remaining 6 tablespoons Parmesan, egg yolks, egg, and salt in a medium mixing basin.
3. Cook the pasta for 1 minute in hot water, stirring periodically. Cook for 1 minute more after adding the spinach and peas, or until the pasta is cooked. 1/4 cup of the cooking water should be set aside. Drain the water and place it in a big mixing basin.
4. Whisk in the saved cooking water slowly into the egg mixture. Toss the spaghetti with tongs as you gradually add the mixture. Serve with the remaining breadcrumb mixture on top.

Nutrition Facts: Calories: 430 | Carbohydrates: 52 g | Protein: 13 g | Fat: 1 g | Cholesterol: 10 mg

278. SAUTÉED BROCCOLI WITH PEANUT SAUCE

Prep Time: 15 minutes
Cook Time: 15 minutes
Total Time: 30 minutes
Servings: 6

Ingredients:
- 8 cups broccoli florets (2-inch pieces)
- 2 tablespoons toasted oil
- 4 cup sliced red bell
- ½ cup sliced yellow onion
- 2 medium cloves garlic, chopped
- tablespoons smooth natural peanut butter
- 2 ½ tablespoons reduced-sodium tamari
- 2 tablespoons rice vinegar
- 2 tablespoon light brown sugar
- 2 teaspoon cornstarch

Directions:
1. Bring 1 inch of water to a boil in a big pot with a steamer basket. Cover and simmer until the broccoli is tender-crisp, 3 to 4 minutes.
2. Meanwhile, in a large pan over medium-high heat, heat the oil. Cook, often turning, until the bell pepper, onion, and garlic soften approximately 3 minutes. Cook, constantly stirring, for 3 minutes after adding the steamed broccoli.
3. In a small mixing bowl, combine the peanut butter, tamari, vinegar, sugar, and cornstarch until smooth. Combine with the veggies. Cook, constantly stirring, for 1 minute, or until the sauce thickens.

Nutrition Facts: Calories: 154 | Carbohydrates: 12 g | Protein: 6 g | Fat: 2 g | Cholesterol: 17 mg

279. SPINACH-STRAWBERRY SALAD WITH FETA &

Prep Time: 15 minutes
Cook Time: 15 minutes
Total Time: 30 minutes
Servings: 4

Ingredients:
- 1 ½ tablespoon extra-virgin olive oil
- 2 tablespoon best-quality balsamic vinegar
- 2 teaspoons finely chopped shallot
- ¼ teaspoon salt
- 6 cups baby spinach
- 2 cup sliced strawberries
- ¼ cup crumbled feta cheese
- ¼ cup toasted chopped

Directions:
1. In a large mixing bowl, combine the oil, vinegar, shallot, salt, and pepper. Allow shallots to soften and mellow for 5 to 10 minutes before serving.
2. Toss the spinach, strawberries, feta, and toss to cover with the dressing in a large mixing basin.

Nutrition Facts: Calories: 158 | Carbohydrates: 52 g | Protein: 15g | Fat: 18 g | Cholesterol: 62 mg

280. SALMON-STUFFED AVOCADOS

Prep Time: 15 minutes
Cook Time: 15 minutes
Total Time: 30 minutes
Servings: 4

Ingredients:
- ½ cup nonfat plain Greek yogurt
- ½ cup diced celery
- 2 tablespoons chopped fresh parsley
- 4 tablespoon lime juice
- 3 teaspoons mayonnaise
- 3 teaspoon Dijon mustard
- ⅛ teaspoon salt
- (5 ounces) cans salmon, drained, flaked, skin and bones removed
- 3 avocados
- Chopped chives for garnish

Directions:
1. Combine yogurt, celery, parsley, lime juice, mayonnaise, mustard, salt, and pepper in a medium mixing bowl. Mix in the salmon well.
2. Cut avocados in half lengthwise and remove the pits. Fill a small bowl with roughly 1 tablespoon flesh from each avocado half. With a fork, mash the scooped-out avocado flesh and toss it into the salmon mixture.
3. Fill about 1/4 cup of the salmon mixture into each half of the avocado, mounding it on top of the halves. If desired, garnish with chives.

Nutrition Facts: Calories: 293 | Carbohydrates: 10 g | Protein: 22 g | Fat: 67 g | Cholesterol: 74 mg

281. BEEFLESS TACOS

Prep Time: 20 minutes
Cook Time: 20 minutes
Total Time: 40 minutes
Servings: 4

Ingredients:
- (16 ounces) package extra-firm tofu, drained, crumbled and patted dry
- 2 tablespoons reduced-sodium tamari or soy sauce
- 1 teaspoon chili powder
- ½ teaspoon garlic powder
- ½ teaspoon onion powder
- 2 tablespoon extra-virgin olive oil

- 1 ripe avocado
- 2 tablespoon vegan mayonnaise
- 2 teaspoon lime juice
- Pinch of salt
- ½ cup fresh salsa or pico de gallo
- 2 cups shredded iceberg lettuce
- 8 corn or flour tortillas, warmed
- Pickled radishes for garnish

Directions:
1. Combine the tofu, tamari (or soy sauce), chili powder, garlic powder, and onion powder in a medium mixing bowl. Heat the oil in a large nonstick skillet over medium-high heat. Cook, stirring occasionally, for 8 to 10 minutes, or until the tofu mixture is thoroughly browned.
2. Meanwhile, mash the avocado, mayonnaise, lime juice, and salt in a separate bowl until smooth.
3. Serve the taco "meat" in tortillas with avocado crema, salsa (or pico de gallo), and lettuce. If desired, top with pickled radishes.

Nutrition Facts: Calories: 350 | Carbohydrates: 62 g | Protein: 28 g | Fat: 10 g | Cholesterol: 63 mg

282. AVOCADO PESTO

Prep Time: 10 minutes
Cook Time: 5 minutes
Total Time: 15 minutes
Servings: 16

Ingredients:
- 2 large bunch fresh basil
- 2 ripe avocados
- ½ cup or hemp s
- 3 tablespoons lemon juice
- 1 cloves garlic
- ½ teaspoon fine sea salt
- ½ cup extra-virgin olive oil

Directions:
1. Remove the basil leaves from the stems and place them in a food processor with the avocados (or hemp seeds), lemon juice, garlic, and salt; pulse until finely chopped. Add the oil and mix until thick paste forms. Season to taste.

Note: Refrigerate for up to 5 days after placing a piece of plastic wrap immediately on the surface to avoid browning.

Nutrition Facts: Calories: 126 | Carbohydrates: 3 g | Protein: 1 g | Fat: 1 g | Cholesterol: 64 mg

283. MEDITERRANEAN CHICKPEA QUINOA BOWL

Prep Time: 20 minutes
Cook Time: 20 minutes
Total Time: 40 minutes
Servings: 3

Ingredients:
- (7 ounces) jar roasted reds, rinsed
- ¼ cup slivered almonds
- 4 tablespoons extra-virgin olive oil, divided
- 2 small clove garlic, minced
- 2 teaspoon paprika
- ½ teaspoon ground cumin
- ¼ teaspoon crushed red (optional)
- ¼ cup Kalamata olives, chopped
- ¼ cup finely chopped red onion
- (15 ounces) can chickpeas, rinsed
- 2 cup diced cucumber
- ¼ cup crumbled feta cheese
- 3 tablespoons finely chopped fresh parsley

Directions:
1. In a small food blender, combine the s, almonds, 2 tablespoons oil, garlic, paprika, cumin, and crushed red pepper (if using). Puree until the mixture is pretty smooth.
2. Combine the quinoa, olives, red onion, and the remaining 2 tablespoons oil in a medium mixing bowl.

3. Divide the quinoa mixture into four dishes and top with chickpeas, cucumber, and red sauce. Garnish with feta and parsley if desired.

Note: Prepare the red sauce (Step 1) and the quinoa (Step 2) separately and chill in separate containers. Assemble only minutes before serving.

Nutrition Facts: Calories: 479 | Carbohydrates: 39 g | Protein: 65 g | Fat: 33 g | Cholesterol: 105 mg

284. PROSCIUTTO PIZZA WITH ARUGULA

Prep Time: 20 minutes
Cook Time: 15 minutes
Total Time: 35 minutes
Servings: 4

Ingredients:
- 2 pound pizza dough, preferably whole-wheat
- 2 tablespoons extra-virgin olive oil, divided
- 3 clove garlic, minced
- 2 cup part-skim shredded mozzarella cheese
- 2 cup fresh kernels
- 3 ounce very thinly sliced prosciutto, torn into 1-inch pieces
- 1 ½ cups arugula
- ½ cup torn fresh basil

Directions:
1. Preheat the grill to medium-high heat. (Alternatively, see Tips if you want to bake.)
2. Roll out the dough into a 12-inch oval on a lightly floured board. Place on a large baking sheet that has been lightly floured. In a small dish, combine 1 tablespoon oil and garlic. To the grill, add the dough, garlic oil, cheese, and prosciutto.
3. Lubricate the grill rack (see Tips). Place the crust on the grill. Grill the dough for 1 to 2 minutes, or until puffed and lightly browned.
4. Spread the garlic oil over the top of the crust. Serve with the cheese and prosciutto on top. Cover the grill for 2 to 3 minutes more, or until the cheese is melted and the crust is gently browned on the bottom. Place the pizza back on the baking pan.
5. Garnish the pizza with arugula, basil, and. Drizzle the remaining 1 tablespoon oil over the top.

Note: Is there no grill? Not a problem! Place the crust on a large greased baking sheet, drizzle with garlic oil, then top with cheese and prosciutto. Bake at 450°F for 18 to 20 minutes, or until the crust is brown on the bottom and the cheese is melted. Garnish with arugula, basil, and. Drizzle the remaining 1 tablespoon oil over the top.
To oil your hot grill rack, wet a paper towel in vegetable oil and brush it over the rack with tongs. (Avoid using cooking spray on a hot grill.)

Nutrition Facts: Calories: 354 | Carbohydrates: 72 g | Protein: 17 g | Fat: 30 g | Cholesterol: 726 mg

285. TEX-MEX PASTA SALAD

Prep Time: 10 minutes
Cook Time: 15 minutes
Total Time: 35 minutes
Servings: 1

Ingredients:
- 2 tablespoon tomatillo salsa
- 2 tablespoon low-fat plain Greek yogurt
- 1 cup cherry tomatoes, halved
- ¾ cup chopped red bell
- ¾ cup of frozen shelled edamame (4 oz.), cooked according to package directions and also drained and cooled
- ½ cup of cooked orzo, preferably whole-wheat, cooled
- ¼ cup of chopped red onion
- 2 tablespoons shredded Jack cheese
- ⅛ teaspoon salt
- Hot sauce, to taste
- 2 tablespoon toasted pepitas (see Tip)

- Lime wedge, for serving

Directions:
1. Combine the salsa and yogurt in a small mixing dish. set aside
2. Combine the tomatoes, bell pepper, edamame, orzo, onion, and cheese in a mixing bowl. Toss in the salt, pepper, and salsa dressing to mix. Season with spicy sauce to taste, top with pepitas, and serve with a slice of lime, if preferred.

Note: Pepitas are pumpkin seeds, but they are not the same as the s you scrape out of your Halloween pumpkin: they originate from pumpkin types that generate seeds without a thick outer shell. Pepitas may be found in bulk bins at natural food stores and major supermarkets, as well as online at.com and elsewhere. To raise a glass: Heat the pepitas in a small saucepan over medium heat. Cook, often stirring, for 1 to 2 minutes, or until lightly browned. To make ahead, cook the pasta up to 1 day ahead of time and chill it.

Nutrition Facts: Calories: 403 | Carbohydrates: 27 g | Protein: 51 g | Fat: 36 g | Cholesterol: 128 mg

286. BARBECUE PULLED JACKFRUIT SANDWICHES

Prep Time: 20 minutes
Cook Time: 25 minutes
Total Time: 45 minutes
Servings: 4

Ingredients:
- ½ cup ketchup
- 3 tablespoons molasses
- 3 tablespoons cider vinegar, divided
- 2 teaspoon vegan Worcestershire sauce
- 2 teaspoon Dijon mustard
- 1 teaspoon hot sauce, or to taste
- ½ teaspoon onion powder
- green jackfruit in brine (20 oz.) washed and shredded
- 2 tablespoons vegan mayonnaise
- ⅛ teaspoon salt
- 3 cups coleslaw mix
- 2 whole-wheat buns, toasted

Directions:
1. In a medium saucepan, combine ketchup, molasses, 1 tablespoon vinegar, Worcestershire, mustard, spicy sauce, and onion powder. Bring to a simmer over medium heat and cook for 5 minutes, stirring occasionally. Cook, stirring constantly, until the jackfruit is cooked through, approximately 5 minutes longer.
2. In a medium mixing bowl, combine mayonnaise, the remaining 2 tablespoons vinegar, and salt. Toss in the coleslaw mix to coat. On the bottom of each bun, spread 1/2 cup of the jackfruit mixture. 2/3 cup slaw on top of the bun top

Nutrition Facts: Calories: 309 | Carbohydrates: 52 g | Protein: 58 g | Fat: 10 g | Cholesterol: 26 mg

287. CHERRY TOMATO & GARLIC PASTA

Prep Time: 20 minutes
Cook Time: 20 minutes
Total Time: 40 minutes
Servings: 5

Ingredients:
- 8 oz whole-wheat penne pasta
- 2 tablespoons extra-virgin olive oil
- 6 cloves garlic, peeled
- 2 cups cherry tomatoes
- 2 medium yellow squash, halved and sliced 1/4 inch thick
- ¾ teaspoon salt
- 1 cup chopped fresh basil
- 3 cup pearl-size or mini mozzarella balls (about 4 oz)
- ¼ cup finely grated Parmesan cheese

Directions:

1. A big pot of water should be brought to a boil. Cook the pasta according to the package guidelines. Set aside 1/4 cup of the cooking water, then drain the pasta and cover to keep warm.
2. Meanwhile, in a large nonstick skillet over medium-high heat, heat the oil. Reduce the heat to medium and simmer, constantly stirring, until the garlic softens and turns light yellow, approximately 3 minutes. Cook, occasionally stirring, until the squash softens and the tomatoes begin to burst, about 4 to 5 minutes. Mash the garlic lightly with the back of a spoon. Turn off the heat.
3. Toss together the pasta, leftover cooking water, basil, and mozzarella in a large mixing bowl. Serve with Parmesan cheese on top.

Nutrition Facts: Calories: 385 | Carbohydrates: 48 g | Protein: 65 g | Fat: 5 g | Cholesterol: 92 mg

CHAPTER 14: SNACKS (FIBER-RICH)

288. ZUCCHINI-CHICKPEA VEGGIE BURGERS WITH TAHINI-RANCH SAUCE

Prep Time: 25 minutes
Cook Time: 25 minutes
Total Time: 50 minutes
Servings: 4

Ingredients:
- 4 tablespoons tahini, divided
- 3 tablespoon lemon juice
- 2 teaspoons white miso, divided
- 1 ¼ teaspoons onion powder, divided
- 1 ¼ teaspoon garlic powder, divided
- 1 cup of water
- 2 teaspoon chopped fresh chives plus 2 tablespoons, divided
- (15 ounces) can no-salt-added chickpeas, rinsed
- 2 teaspoon ground cumin
- ¼ teaspoon salt
- ¼ cup fresh parsley leaves
- ½ cup shredded zucchini
- ⅓ cup old-fashioned rolled oats
- 2 tablespoon extra-virgin olive oil
- 1 whole-grain hamburger buns, toasted
- 1 cup packed fresh arugula
- 2 slices tomato

Directions:
1. In a small mixing bowl, combine 2 tablespoons tahini, lemon juice, 1 teaspoon miso, 1/2 teaspoon onion powder, 1/4 teaspoon garlic powder, and 1/4 teaspoon. Whisk in the water gradually until the mixture is smooth. 1 teaspoon chives, stirred in Place aside.
2. In a food processor, combine chickpeas, cumin, salt, and the remaining 2 tablespoons tahini, 2 teaspoons miso, 1 teaspoon garlic powder, 1 teaspoon, and 3/4 teaspoon onion powder. Pulse until a gritty mixture develops that holds together when pushed, stopping once or twice to wipe down the edges. Pulse in the parsley and remaining 2 tablespoons chives until the herbs are finely chopped and integrated into the mixture. Transfer to a mixing basin.
3. To remove excess moisture, squeeze zucchini in a clean kitchen towel. Add the zucchini and oats to the chickpea mixture and mash together with your fingertips. Form the mixture into four patties.
4. In a large nonstick skillet over medium-high heat, heat the oil. Cook until the patties are brown and beginning to crisp, 4 to 5 minutes. Cook until golden brown on the other side, 2 to 4 minutes more.
5. To serve, top the burgers with the tahini-ranch sauce, arugula, and tomato slices.

Note: The burger patties and tahini ranch sauce can be prepared ahead of time. Prepare through Step 3; refrigerate for up to 24 hours, covered individually.

Nutrition Facts: Calories: 373 | Carbohydrates: 48 g | Protein: 52 g | Fat: 48 g | Cholesterol: 90 mg

289. CHICKPEA BURGERS & TAHINI SAUCE

Prep Time: 10 minutes
Cook Time: 15 minutes
Total Time: 25 minutes
Servings: 3

Ingredients:
- Chickpea burgers
- 19-ounce can chickpeas, rinsed
- 4 scallions, trimmed and sliced

- 3 egg
- 2 tablespoons all-purpose flour
- 1 tablespoon chopped fresh oregano
- ½ teaspoon ground cumin
- ¼ teaspoon salt
- 2 tablespoons extra-virgin olive oil
- 6-1/2-inch whole-wheat pitas, halved and warmed, if desired
- Tahini sauce
- ½ cup low-fat plain yogurt
- 1 tablespoon tahini, (see Ingredient note)
- 2 tablespoon lemon juice
- ⅓ cup chopped flat-leaf parsley
- ¼ teaspoon salt

Directions:
1. Combine chickpeas, scallions, egg, flour, oregano, cumin, and salt in a food blender. Pulse until a gritty mixture develops that holds together when pushed, stopping once or twice to wipe down the edges. (The mixture will be somewhat wet.) Form the mixture into four patties.
2. Heat the oil in a large nonstick skillet over medium-high heat. Cook for 4 to 5 minutes, or until the patties are golden brown and crisp. Cook for another 2 to 4 minutes on the other side, or until golden brown.
3. To make the sauce and serve it, follow these steps: Meanwhile, in a medium mixing bowl, combine the yogurt, tahini, lemon juice, parsley, and salt. If preferred, warm pita bread. On top of the pita halves, serve the burgers with the sauce.

Note: Refrigerate the uncooked burger mixture and tahini sauce for up to 2 days, covered.

Nutrition Facts: Calories: 400 | Carbohydrates: 54 g | Protein: 27 g | Fat: 19 g | Cholesterol: 130 mg

290. **FALAFEL BURGERS**

Prep Time: 30 minutes
Cook Time: 60 minutes
Total Time: 90 minutes
Servings: 4

Ingredients:
- ½ cup coarsely chopped onion
- 3 cloves garlic, crushed
- 2 medium jalapeño , ed and coarsely chopped
- ¾ cup fresh cilantro and/or parsley leaves
- (15 ounce) can no-salt-added chickpeas, rinsed
- 2 teaspoons ground cumin
- 1 teaspoon ground coriander
- ¼ teaspoon baking soda
- ¼ teaspoon salt
- ⅓ cup dry whole-wheat breadcrumbs or gluten-free breadcrumbs
- 2 tablespoon extra-virgin olive oil
- 1 whole-wheat or gluten-free burger buns, split and toasted

Directions:
1. Combine the onion, garlic, jalapeo, and cilantro (or parsley) in a mixing bowl and pulse until evenly diced. Combine chickpeas, cumin, coriander, baking soda, and salt in a mixing bowl. Process until everything is thoroughly mixed. Transfer to a medium mixing bowl. Mix in the breadcrumbs. Refrigerate for 20 minutes, covered. (This permits extra moisture to be absorbed by the breadcrumbs.)
2. Preheat the oven to 375°F. Form the chickpea mixture into four 3-inch-diameter patties, using a generous 1/3 cup each burger.
3. In a large skillet over medium heat, heat the oil. Cook until the patties are brown and crispy, about 4 minutes per side. Transfer the patties to a baking sheet and bake for 15 minutes, or until cooked through and slightly puffed. Place the patties on buns and serve.

Nutrition Facts: Calories: 267 | Carbohydrates: 17 g | Protein: 10 g | Fat: 0.9 g | Cholesterol: 85 mg

291. MUSHROOM-QUINOA VEGGIE BURGERS WITH SPECIAL SAUCE

Prep Time: 25 minutes
Cook Time: 60 minutes
Total Time: 85 minutes
Servings: 3

Ingredients:
- 2 large portobello mushrooms, gills removed, roughly chopped
- 2 cup no-salt-added canned black beans, rinsed
- 2 tablespoons unsalted creamy almond butter
- 2 tablespoons canola mayonnaise, divided
- ¾ teaspoon smoked paprika
- ¾ teaspoon garlic powder, divided
- ½ teaspoon salt
- ½ cup cooked quinoa
- ¼ cup old-fashioned rolled oats
- 2 tablespoon ketchup
- 2 teaspoon Dijon mustard
- 3 tablespoon extra-virgin olive oil
- 2 whole-wheat hamburger buns, toasted
- 2 leaves green-leaf lettuce, halved
- 2 slices tomato
- 1 thin slices red onion

Directions:
1. In a food processor, combine the mushroom, black beans, almond butter, 1 tablespoon mayonnaise, paprika, 1/2 teaspoon garlic powder, and salt. Pulse until a gritty mixture develops that holds together when pushed, stopping once or twice to wipe down the edges. Transfer to a mixing bowl and toss in the quinoa and oats. 1 hour in the refrigerator
2. Meanwhile, in a separate bowl, mix together ketchup, mustard, the remaining 2 tablespoons mayonnaise, and 1/4 teaspoon garlic powder until smooth.
3. Form the mushroom mixture into four patties.
4. In a large grill pan or nonstick skillet, heat the oil over medium-high heat. Cook until the patties are brown and beginning to crisp, 4 to 5 minutes. Cook for another 2 to 4 minutes, or until golden brown on the opposite side.
5. Serve the burgers with the special sauce, lettuce, tomato, and onion on buns.

Nutrition Facts: Calories: 395 | Carbohydrates: 62 g | Protein: 10 g | Fat: 63 g | Cholesterol: 50 mg

292. CILANTRO BEAN BURGERS WITH CREAMY AVOCADO-LIME SLAW

Prep Time: 45 minutes
Cook Time: 45 minutes
Total Time: 90 minutes
Servings: 5

Ingredients:
- (15 ounce) can no-salt-added black beans, rinsed
- 2 cloves garlic, minced, divided
- ½ teaspoon ground cumin
- ½ teaspoon salt, divided
- ¼ cup crushed tortilla chips or panko breadcrumbs
- ¼ cup quick-cooking oats
- 2 tablespoons toasted pumpkin s, chopped
- Two tablespoons of chopped fresh cilantro plus 1/2 cup, divided
- 2 large egg, lightly beaten
- ¼ cup low-fat plain Greek yogurt
- ½ avocado
- 1 teaspoon lime zest
- 2 tablespoons lime juice
- 1 cup of water

- 2 cups shredded cabbage (green and/or red)
- 2 teaspoons olive oil
- 3 whole-wheat buns, halved and toasted

Directions:
1. In a medium mixing dish, combine the beans, half the garlic, cumin, and 1/4 teaspoon salt. With a fork, mash the beans until they are completely mashed. Mix in the crumbled chips (or panko), oats, pumpkin seeds, 2 tablespoons cilantro, and the egg.
2. Divide the ingredients into four equal halves and form them into patties. Refrigerate for 30 minutes before cooking on a platter.
3. Meanwhile, in a blender or food processor, mix the remaining 1/2 cup cilantro, remaining garlic, yogurt, avocado, lime juice, and water. Blend until smooth. Transfer to a large mixing bowl. Combine the lime zest and the remaining 1/4 teaspoon salt in a mixing bowl. Toss in the cabbage to mix.
4. In a large nonstick saucepan over medium heat, heat the oil. Cook for 6 minutes after adding the burgers. Turn them over, decrease the heat to medium, cover, and cook for 5 to 6 minutes more, or until golden brown and warmed through. Serve the burgers on buns with 1/4 cup cabbage slaw on top. Serve the rest of the slaw on the side.

Nutrition Facts: Calories: 368 | Carbohydrates: 54 g | Protein: 20 g | Fat: 11 g | Cholesterol: 30 mg

293. ROSEMARY ALMOND FLOUR PUMPKIN BREAD

Prep Time: 15 minutes
Cook Time: 45 minutes
Total Time: 60 minutes
Servings: 10

Ingredients:
- 3/4 cup pumpkin puree
- ½ cup of avocado oil or olive oil
- 3 large eggs
- 3 teaspoon apple cider vinegar (or white vinegar)
- 2 cup blanched almond flour
- 1/4 cup tapioca flour or arrowroot flour
- 1/4 cup raw sugar or monk fruit sugar
- 2 teaspoon baking soda
- pinch of allspice or nutmeg
- 1/2 teaspoon kosher salt
- pinch black
- 2 Tablespoon fresh rosemary sprigs (or 3 teaspoons dried rosemary, divided)
- 1/4 cup raw or roasted pumpkin s (divided)

Directions:
1. Preheat the oven to 350 degrees F. Line a 9-inch bread pan, an 8-inch loaf pan, or two mini loaf pans with parchment paper (see notes). Grease or oil the pans' inside.
2. Combine the pumpkin, eggs, oil, and vinegar in a mixing dish. Gently whisk or combine the items with a spoon until smooth.
3. Sift together the almond flour, tapioca flour, sugar, baking soda, spices, and salt in a separate bowl. Set aside the pumpkins and rosemary sprigs.
4. Gently fold a portion of the flour mixture into the wet ingredients until the batter is smooth. Repeat this step until all of the flour has been well mixed with the wet ingredients.
5. One teaspoon fresh rosemary or Two teaspoons dry rosemary and 2 to 3 tablespoons pumpkin puree. Save the leftover s for garnishing.
6. Pour the batter into the loaf pan that has been prepared (or 2 smaller mini loaf pans).
7. On top of the batter, scatter the pumpkin seeds and additional rosemary.

8. 40-45 minutes in the oven After 30 minutes, check the bread for doneness. If the center is still not done, cover with foil and bake for another 5-10 minutes, or until golden brown and a toothpick inserted into the middle comes out clean.
9. Allow the bread to cool in the pan after removing it from the oven. After the bread has cooled, take it from the pan and slice it or store it later.

Nutrition Facts: Calories: 238 | Carbohydrates: 6 g | Protein: 9 g | Fat: 2 g | Cholesterol: 10 mg

294. ORANGE ZUCCHINI BREAD

Prep Time: 10 minutes
Cook Time: 60 minutes
Total Time: 70 minutes
Servings: 10

Ingredients:
- 2 1/4 cup almond flour
- 1/4 cup coconut flour
- 1/2 tablespoon salt
- 2 tablespoon baking powder
- ½ cup of coconut sugar or raw sugar
- 1/2 tablespoon ground cinnamon and/or ginger
- medium zucchini (grated, water extracted)
- 1/2 cup fresh orange juice (divided)
- 4 eggs room temp
- 1/3 to 1/2 c coconut milk or almond milk (regular cream may be substituted)
- 2 tablespoon melted coconut oil
- 1 ½ tablespoon vanilla
- Orange slices to top
- Optional orange ginger glaze – not strict paleo, sugar-free option
- 1/2 cup powdered sugar
- ½ tablespoon – ¼ cup orange juice
- 2 tablespoon melted butter or coconut oil
- 1/4 tablespoon ground ginger
- dash of orange zest or orange peel

Directions:

1. Preheat the oven to 350 degrees Fahrenheit. Line a loaf pan with parchment paper and brush the sides with oil. 95°F or 84°F for denser bread
2. In a small mixing bowl, sift the almond flour/coconut flour, salt, baking powder, and cinnamon; whisk in the sugar and mix until mixed. Set aside.
3. Place the zucchini on a dish or in a bowl and grate it. Using a paper towel, press the grated zucchini to remove as much water as possible. Alternatively, wrap the zucchini in a towel and squeeze out the excess water. Return to the bowl.
4. Next, whisk or combine the eggs, milk, and 1/3 cup orange juice (in a blender or hand mixer). Save the remaining 1/4 cup for a glaze if desired.
5. Mix the wet and dry ingredients in a separate bowl. If the batter is too dry, add a little extra milk.
6. Mix in the melted coconut oil and vanilla extract. Finally, fold in the zucchini.
7. Place the batter in a loaf or bread pan. The batter will be thick because of the coconut flour, so you may need to use a spatula to smooth it out in the pan. On top, arrange thinly sliced orange slices.
8. Bake for 50-60 minutes on the center rack of the oven.
9. Check the center with a knife or toothpick after 45 minutes to ensure it is clean. The bread might take up to 70 minutes to bake, depending on the oven. If the bread takes longer than 50 minutes, cover with foil and continue baking until the middle is firm.
10. Remove the baking sheet from the oven and put it aside to cool. Spread the optional glaze over the top before slicing, or leave it off and slice as is.

For The Optional Ginger Glaze
1. In a small mixing basin, whisk together all of the ingredients until smooth. See the post for a link to a sugar-free powdered sugar alternative.
2. Drizzle the glaze over the bread before serving, or over each slice.

3. If not in use, place it in the refrigerator. If you're using coconut oil, you'll need to warm it up a little before putting it in the fridge.

Nutrition Facts: Calories: 268 | Carbohydrates: 17 g | Protein: 6 g | Fat: 10 g | Cholesterol: 70 mg

295. **NUT AND BREAD**

Prep Time: 10 minutes
Cook Time: 35 minutes
Total Time: 45 minutes
Servings: 12

Ingredients:
- 5 large eggs (see notes)
- 1/3 cup olive oil (see notes)
- 2 tablespoon white or apple cider vinegar
- 1/3 to 1 1/2 cups blanched almond flour (145 g)
- 1/2 tablespoon kosher salt
- dash of black
- 2 tablespoon spice(s) of choice – OPTIONAL (garlic, rosemary, Italian, etc.)
- 3 tablespoon poppy s, plus extra for topping
- 2 tablespoon tapioca flour/starch
- 1/2 tablespoon baking soda
- 1/4 cup flax meal or ground chia

For Topping
- Pumpkin s
- hemp s
- poppy s

Directions:
1. Preheat oven to 350 degrees Fahrenheit. Using parchment paper, line a 9x5-inch loaf pan. Set aside.
2. Whisk together the eggs, oil, and vinegar in a small bowl.
3. Add the dry ingredients to a large mixing bowl and whisk to incorporate. Combine the wet and dry ingredients and thoroughly combine.
4. Fill prepared loaf pan halfway with batter and top with pumpkin, hemp, and poppy seeds.
5. Bake for 20 minutes, then uncover and bake for another 15-20 minutes, or until brown and a knife inserted into the middle of the loaf comes out clean.
6. Remove from oven and cool for 10 minutes in the pan before putting out onto a cooling rack.
7. If preferred, slice the loaf, then cover it in foil or plastic wrap and keep it in an airtight container. Keep refrigerated for up to 7 days or freeze for up to 3 months.

Nutrition Facts: Calories: 175 | Carbohydrates: 3 g | Protein: 5 g | Fat: 5 g | Cholesterol: 180 mg

296. **PUMPKIN STUFFED DOUGH BALLS**

Prep Time: 10 minutes
Cook Time: 20 minutes
Total Time: 30 minutes
Servings: 7

Ingredients:
For the dough
- 1/2 cup of cassava flour (or GF multi purpose flour)
- 2 cup coconut or almond milk
- 1/2 tablespoon baking soda
- pinch of sea salt
- 2 tablespoon sweetener (coconut sugar or honey works)
- brush dough with melted butter or oil before baking

Fillings
- Pureed pumpkin (unsweetened).
- 1/2 thumb size cube of jack cheese or dairy-free cheese of choice (in each dough ball).
- A pinch of garlic salt
- Any additional herbs or savory stuffing of your choosing

- Butter made from nuts (1 or 2 tablespoons in each dough ball).
- A pinch of cinnamon
- 1/2 tablespoon maple syrup or honey

Directions:
1. Preheat the oven to 350 degrees Fahrenheit.
2. In a mixing bowl, combine the flour, sugar, salt, and baking soda.
3. Microwave your milk for 1 or 2 minutes.
4. Gradually put in the hot milk and combine the mixture until it becomes a thick dough-like batter.
5. Scoop out a piece the size of your palm and roll it into a ball.
6. Should yield around 7-8 balls.
7. Press the ball flat, then insert your filling of choice. A small spoonful of pumpkin, followed by your additional ingredient of choice.
8. So, for the sweet dough balls, add 1 tablespoon nut butter, a tiny spoonful or less of pumpkin, a sprinkle of cinnamon, and a drizzle (1/2 tablespoon) of honey.
9. Next, cut the dough ball in your palm to seal the filling.
10. Place on a baking pan upside down.
11. Rep the filling for the remaining dough balls.
12. Brush each dough ball with a little coconut oil or butter after it's on the baking sheet.
13. Bake for 15–20 minutes, or until the dough is golden brown.
14. For the sweet dough balls, I sprinkled coconut sugar on top before baking.

Nutrition Facts: Calories: 382 | Carbohydrates: 19 g | Protein: 58 g | Fat: 40 g | Cholesterol: 28 mg

297. **HOMEMADE GRAHAM CRACKERS**

Prep Time: 10 minutes
Cook Time: 60 minutes
Total Time: 70 minutes
Servings: 8

Ingredients:
- 1--1/2 cup (150 grams) of gluten-free oat flour (see this recipe for making oat flour)
- 1/4 cup (30 grams) of blanched fine almond flour
- Three teaspoons of baking powder
- 1/2 teaspoon of baking soda
- 1/8 – 1/4 teaspoon of salt
- 1/3 – 1/2 cup of raw sugar (or granulated sweetener of choice)
- 1/4 teaspoon of cinnamon
- 4 Tablespoons of cold butter, chopped (vegan butter may be substituted)
- 6 Tablespoons of cold non-dairy milk
- 2 Tablespoons of honey (or maple syrup for vegan option)
- 1/2 teaspoon of vanilla extract

Directions:
1. Preheat the oven to 350 degrees Fahrenheit. Set aside a big sheet pan or rimless cookie sheet lined with parchment paper.
2. Whisk/sift the oat flour, almond flour, baking powder, baking soda, and salt in a large mixing basin or stand mixer bowl. Whisk in the sugar and cinnamon until combined.
3. Set the stand mixer to dough paddle mode. In place of a stand mixer, a food processor can be used (see notes).
4. Add the chopped cold butter to the stand mixer on medium speed. Mix until a mealy flour forms.
5. Then, add the cool milk, honey, and vanilla extract. Mix on medium to medium-high until everything is incorporated.
6. Take the bowl out of the stand mixer. Hand-knead the dough until it forms a softball. To chill the dough, wrap it in plastic wrap and place it in the fridge for 1-2 hours or in the freezer for 15 minutes.
7. Place the cold dough on a well-floured surface or wax paper dusted with oat flour.
8. Cover the dough with plastic wrap. Then, using a rolling pin, spread out the dough into a large rectangle about 1/8-inch thick.

9. Flip the dough onto the baking pan with care. Using a sharp knife or pastry cutter, cut the dough into 3-inch by 3-inch squares. With your fingertips, remove any excess dough.
10. Prick the crackers with a fork (score). Prick is just halfway through. If desired, top the cookies with additional raw cane sugar.
11. Place the baking sheet in the oven's center rack. Bake for 7 minutes, then flip the pan and bake for another 7-8 minutes (total time 13-15 minutes), or until the crackers are golden and firm to the touch.
12. Allow the crackers to cool before cutting them apart.
13. If not dried out, they will be crisp for a few days before softening.

Nutrition Facts: Calories: 129 | Carbohydrates: 18 g | Protein: 38 g | Fat: 20 g | Cholesterol: 47 mg

298. APPLE AND OAT PANCAKES

Prep Time: 5 minutes
Cook Time: 25 minutes
Total Time: 30 minutes
Servings: 1

Ingredients:
- 2 cup oat flour
- 6 oz apple (170 g)
- 2 cup water
- One tablespoon baking powder
- 2 ½ tablespoon vanilla extract (optional)
- Two tablespoon maple syrup (optional)
- 1/3 tablespoon spices (optional)

Directions:
1. Combine all of the ingredients and blended them.
2. Blend for a total of 15 seconds.
3. Allow for a 15-minute resting period for the pancake batter.
4. In a medium saucepan, heat one teaspoon of oil over low heat. (Alternatively, use a nonstick pan.)
5. Cook the pancakes until golden brown on both sides.
6. Allow the pancakes to cool fully before sprinkling them with apples, maple syrup, salted caramel sauce, or peanut butter.

Nutrition Facts: Calories: 55 | Carbohydrates: 10 g | Protein: 13 g | Fat: 1 g | Cholesterol: 10 mg

299. BLACKBERRY QUINOA BREAKFAST BOWL

Prep Time: 5 minutes
Cook Time: 15 minutes
Total Time: 20 minutes
Servings: 4

Ingredients:
- ½ cup uncooked quinoa rinsed well underwater
- ¾ cup water
- 1 ½ cup unsweetened almond milk
- Two teaspoon cinnamon
- Two teaspoon vanilla extract
- One tablespoon maple syrup
- Handful of almonds
- Two teaspoons flax s
- ¼ cup blackberries
- Dried rosebuds for garnish

Directions:
1. Bring quinoa & water to a boil in a small saucepan. Reduce the heat to low and cook, covered, for 15 to 20 minutes, or until the water has evaporated. Allow it to cool.
2. Combine almond milk, cinnamon, vanilla essence, and maple syrup in a mixing bowl.
3. Divide the cooked quinoa among the bowls and top with the milk mixture. There is no specific measurement for this; simply pour as much as you wish.
4. Almonds, flax seeds, blackberries, and dried rosebuds can be sprinkled on top.

Nutrition Facts: Calories: 170 | Carbohydrates: 21 g | Protein: 38 g | Fat: 40 g | Cholesterol: 0 mg

300. PROTEIN MUFFINS (5 INGREDIENTS:!)

Prep Time: 5 minutes
Cook Time: 10 minutes
Total Time: 15 minutes
Servings: 8

Ingredients:
- Two scoops of vanilla protein powder 64-67 grams
- Two teaspoon baking powder
- 1/2 cup almond flour
- ½ cup peanut butter or any nut or butter
- 2 cup unsweetened applesauce
- 1/2 cup chocolate chips optional

Directions:
1. Preheat the oven to 180/350 degrees Fahrenheit. Set aside eight muffin liners and a muffin pan.
2. Add the dry ingredients to a large mixing bowl and well combine. Mix in the peanut butter and unsweetened applesauce until well mixed. Fold in the chocolate chips.
3. Bake for 10-12 minutes, or until a skewer comes out largely clean, after dividing the mixture among the muffin liners.
4. Allow the muffins to rest for 5 minutes in the oven before transferring to a wire rack to cool fully.

Nutrition Facts: Calories: 192 | Carbohydrates: 37 g | Protein: 47 g | Fat: 29 g | Cholesterol: 10 mg

YOUR 30-DAY MEAL PLAN

How to Meal-Prep for Weeks of Meals:
A little preparation at the start of the week goes a long way toward making the rest of the week run smoothly.

Day (1104 calories)				
Breakfast	**A.M. Snack**	**Lunch**	**P.M. Snack**	**Dinner**
Apple and pear pita pockets	Zucchini-chickpea veggie burgers with tahini-ranch sauce	Ultimate green detox juice	Lemon ricotta cake	Bacon & balsamic tomatoes
Day 2 (1132 calories)				
Breakfast	**A.M. Snack**	**Lunch**	**P.M. Snack**	**Dinner**
Apple raisin pancakes	Chickpea burgers & tahini sauce	Raw cherry-apple pie	Sweet fried plantains	Chocolate-chipotle sirloin steak
Day 3 (1093 calories)				
Breakfast	**A.M. Snack**	**Lunch**	**P.M. Snack**	**Dinner**
Banana and blueberry fritters	Falafel burgers	Southern shrub	Mango pudding	Cheese sauce
Day 4 (1264 calories)				
Breakfast	**A.M. Snack**	**Lunch**	**P.M. Snack**	**Dinner**
Sweet potato pancakes	Mushroom-quinoa veggie burgers with special sauce	Rosemary lime kiss	French chocolate silk pie	Crock pot cream cheese chicken
Day 5 (976 calories)				
Breakfast	**A.M. Snack**	**Lunch**	**P.M. Snack**	**Dinner**
Spinach pancakes	Cilantro bean burgers with creamy avocado-lime slaw	Ruby red punch	Peanut butter oatmeal chocolate chip cookies	Potatoes
Day 6 (817 calories)				
Breakfast	**A.M. Snack**	**Lunch**	**P.M. Snack**	**Dinner**
Banana and oat cookies	Rosemary almond flour pumpkin bread	Eggy devils	Banana oatmeal chocolate chip cookies	Peanut butter and jelly pb&j smoothie

		Day 7 (837 calories)		
Breakfast	**A.M. Snack**	**Lunch**	**P.M. Snack**	**Dinner**
Banana pancakes	Orange zucchini bread	Caramel sauced oranges	Larabar snack bar	Chocolate mason jar ice cream
		Day 8 (1054 calories)		
Breakfast	**A.M. Snack**	**Lunch**	**P.M. Snack**	**Dinner**
Lentil spinach pancakes	Nut and bread	Pulled chicken salad	Kulfi indian ice cream	Dry rub ribs
		Day 9 (1185 calories)		
Breakfast	**A.M. Snack**	**Lunch**	**P.M. Snack**	**Dinner**
Chickpea pancakes	Pumpkin stuffed dough balls	Beetroot carrot salad	Easy no-bake key lime pie	Prosciutto & spinach egg cups
		Day 10(1269 calories)		
Breakfast	**A.M. Snack**	**Lunch**	**P.M. Snack**	**Dinner**
Veggie chickpea sticks	Homemade graham crackers	Lemongrass beef	Lemon cheesecake recipe	Easy pea & spinach carbonara
		Day 11 (1114 calories)		
Breakfast	**A.M. Snack**	**Lunch**	**P.M. Snack**	**Dinner**
High-fibre muesli	Dreamy berry parfait with coconut whipped cream, caramel & raw granola clusters	Tropical carrot apple juice	French toast	Sautéed broccoli with peanut sauce
		Day 12 (1164 calories)		
Breakfast	**A.M. Snack**	**Lunch**	**P.M. Snack**	**Dinner**
Mexican bean soup with guacamole	Creamy raspberry, coconut & chia shake	Zesty lemon apple juice	Pineapple orange creamsicle	Spinach-strawberry salad with feta &
		Day 13 (1264 calories)		
Breakfast	**A.M. Snack**	**Lunch**	**P.M. Snack**	**Dinner**

Wholemeal soda bread	Toasted coconut and berry grain	Friendly green juice	Easy peach cobbler recipe with bisquick	Salmon-stuffed avocados
Day 14 (1032 calories)				
Breakfast	A.M. Snack	Lunch	P.M. Snack	Dinner
Scrambled eggs	Coconut almond protein bars	Tropical smoothie (pineapple, papaya, coconut, lime smoothie)	Healthy 5-minute strawberry pineapple sherbet	Beefless tacos
Day 15 (906 calories)				
Breakfast	A.M. Snack	Lunch	P.M. Snack	Dinner
Strawberry breakfast cake	Grain free granola clusters	Chicken broth	Best coconut milk ice cream	Avocado pesto
Day 16 (1492 calories)				
Breakfast	A.M. Snack	Lunch	P.M. Snack	Dinner
Blueberry protein shake	Spiced pumpkin granola	Chicken detox soup	Lemon crinkle cookies	Mediterranean chickpea quinoa bowl
Day 17 (1732 calories)				
Breakfast	A.M. Snack	Lunch	P.M. Snack	Dinner
Chickpea scramble breakfast bowl	Pumpkin pie chia pudding	Banana oat shake	Best no-bake chocolate lasagna	Prosciutto pizza with arugula
Breakfast	A.M. Snack	Lunch	P.M. Snack	Dinner
3-ingredient chocolate cereal	Pumpkin pie butter	Banana-apple smoothie	Easiest healthy watermelon smoothie	Tex-mex pasta salad
Day 19 (942 calories)				
Breakfast	A.M. Snack	Lunch	P.M. Snack	Dinner
Veggie quiche with sweet potato crust	Lemon-blueberry muffins	Berrylicious smoothie	Best orange julius	Barbecue pulled jackfruit sandwiches
Day 20 (1153 calories)				
Breakfast	A.M. Snack	Lunch	P.M. Snack	Dinner

	Blueberry almond oatmeal	Sweet potato casserole with praline topping	Citrus relish	Watermelon	Cherry tomato & garlic pasta

Day 21 (1143 calories)					
Breakfast	A.M. Snack	Lunch	P.M. Snack	Dinner
Granola yogurt breakfast trifle	Skinny loaded stuffed baked potato soup	Red wine sangria recipe	Mango prawn poke bowl	Candied orange peel

Day 22 (1492 calories)				
Breakfast	A.M. Snack	Lunch	P.M. Snack	Dinner
Lime mint smoothie	Tomato potato sausage pesto frittata	Salty dog cocktail	Citrus swordfish	Hot buttered rum

Day 23 (732 calories)				
Breakfast	A.M. Snack	Lunch	P.M. Snack	Dinner
Chicken vegetable pasta soup	Broccoli red egg bites	Rose sangria	Honey-herb chicken	Caramel hot apple cider

Day 24 (711 calories)				
Breakfast	A.M. Snack	Lunch	P.M. Snack	Dinner
Beet carrot soup	Breakfast shrimp egg white muffin cups	White sangria	Red rosemary vinegar	Hot apple cider wassail

Day 25 (912 calories)				
Breakfast	A.M. Snack	Lunch	P.M. Snack	Dinner
Broth braised asparagus	Egg potato bites	Raspberry mojitos with basil	Herb-crusted tilapia	Mango smoothie

Day 26 (808 calories)				
Breakfast	A.M. Snack	Lunch	P.M. Snack	Dinner
Banana bran muffins	Vanilla pear raspberry panna cotta	Stir-fry velveted chicken and vegetables	Blood orange chia pudding	Jugo verde

Day 27 (664 calories)				
Breakfast	A.M. Snack	Lunch	P.M. Snack	Dinner

Orange and cinnamon biscotti	Vanilla soy pudding	Black beans and avocado toasts	Blueberry coconut smoothie bowl	Asian bloody mary cocktail

Day 28 (1293 calories)

Breakfast	A.M. Snack	Lunch	P.M. Snack	Dinner
Chocolate smoothie	Apple and oat pancakes	Packed burrito	Springtime tofu scramble	Agua fresca

Day 29 (1311 calories)

Breakfast	A.M. Snack	Lunch	P.M. Snack	Dinner
Asparagus and bean frittata	Protein muffins	Apples n' oats breakfast smoothie	2 minute flourless english muffin	Southern orangeade

Day 30 (982 calories)

Breakfast	A.M. Snack	Lunch	P.M. Snack	Dinner
Apricot honey oatmeal	Blackberry quinoa breakfast bowl	No bake apricot oat protein bars	Blueberry chia jam	Vodka gummy bears popsicles

CONCLUSION

A high-fiber, high-water diet is usually recommended for diverticulitis. It will ensure that your gastrointestinal tract and system get enough rest, allowing you to recuperate. As soon as you start eating properly, you should see results in a few days.

Water intake is equally important; the usual guideline is that your body will need 1/2 of your weight in oz per day so that a 150-pound person will require 75 oz of water each day. Water coupled with a high fiber diet is required to keep your colon moving properly and reduce the risk of an attack or the formation of further diverticula.

Seeds and nuts should be avoided like the plague! Anything with a husk, such as sesame seeds, should be avoided at all costs. In essence, they will irritate the lining of your colon once again, resulting in the formation of diverticula.

Maize is another item to avoid if at all possible, including any corn-based products such as popcorn or cornflour and tortillas. Chilli peppers and other hot and spicy foods are thought to be very hazardous to diverticulitis sufferers.

If your diverticulitis diet plan allows it, try to consume fruits and vegetables that you like. If you don't like greens, consider eating more fresh fruit instead, and vice versa. Vegetable and fruit seeds are safe to eat for most patients, such as those found in cucumbers and tomatoes.

Foods that are high in fiber. Whole-wheat bread and other whole-grain items are high in dietary fiber. You may also add bran to your food. Uncooked or just lightly cooked legumes, as well as fermented greens (e.g., sauerkraut). Fresh fruit and vegetables should not be peeled; they should be consumed naturally (juices are devoid of fiber). Dried fruit, such as raisins, plums, apricots, and dates, are an excellent source.

Naturally, just as we don't all consume the same kind of meals throughout life, diverticulitis foods to avoid will vary from case to instance. Our unhealthy eating habits and poor nutrition and the poisons that arise from them are the root reasons. It's an excellent time to become interested in health and nutrition if you haven't already guessed.

If you wish to reduce or perhaps eliminate future episodes of diverticulitis, you need to eat the right foods. While antibiotics may frequently alleviate severe pain and suffering in the short term, taking them for an extended length of time can be nearly as hazardous as the illness itself, not to mention that your body will ultimately become resistant to their effects.

Consequently, it is often essential to undergo a hazardous and invasive operation, which may result in a decrease in life quality.

Most people would agree that prevention is preferable to treatment. So, to avoid this illness from infecting your stomach, and in light of the current economic climate, we should pay close attention to our health and take appropriate action. Because it is nearly completely due to a lack of dietary fiber, the best course of treatment is to consume the appropriate meals.

Do Not Go Yet; One Last Thing To Do

If you liked this book or found it useful, I'd appreciate it if you could leave a quick review on Amazon. Your support is greatly appreciated, and I personally read all of the reviews in order to obtain your feedback and improve the book.

Thanks for your help and support!

Recipe Index

CHAPTER 5: BREAKFAST (CLEAR FLUIDS) 39
1. APPLE AND PEAR PITA POCKETS 39
2. BRANDY JAVA ICE 39
3. APPLE RAISIN PANCAKES 39
4. BANANA AND BLUEBERRY FRITTERS 40
5. BANANA AND OAT COOKIES 40
6. BANANA PANCAKES 41
7. SWEET POTATO PANCAKES 41
8. LENTIL SPINACH PANCAKES 42
9. CHICKPEA PANCAKES RECIPE 42
10. VEGGIE CHICKPEA STICKS 43
11. APRICOT HONEY OATMEAL 43
12. ASPARAGUS AND BEAN FRITTATA 44
13. CHOCOLATE SMOOTHIE 44
14. ORANGE AND CINNAMON BISCOTTI 44
15. BANANA BRAN MUFFINS 45
16. BANANA BREAKFAST SMOOTHIE 45
17. SWEET & NUTTY BARS 46
18. HOMEMADE HERBED BISCUITS 46
19. SPINACH VEGETABLE BARLEY BEAN SOUP 46
20. SCD SOUR CREAM RECIPE 47
21. SKINNY PUMPKIN SPICE CHAI LATTE RECIPE 47
22. EASY TOMATO BASIL SOUP 47
23. SUGAR-FREE CHOCOLATE MOUSSE 48
24. BLUEBERRY SMOOTHIE 48
25. KATZ'S MAGIC MINERAL BROTH 49
26. CHILE RELLENO CHICKEN SOUP 49
27. THAI COCONUT CURRY LENTIL SOUP 50
28. LEMON VANILLA BEAN CUSTARD 50
29. POT KETO YOGURT 51
30. BANANA COCONUT CHIA PUDDING 51
31. BANANA PUDDING 52
32. CREAM OF MUSHROOM SOUP 52
33. SUGAR-FREE APPLESAUCE 53
34. APPLE ARUGULA FLATBREAD 53
35. APPLE CHIPS 54
36. SUGAR-FREE APPLE CRISP 55
37. CHOCOLATE NICE CREAM 55
38. HEALTHY WATERMELON POPSICLES 56
39. SPINACH MANGO VEGAN POPSICLES 56
40. MANGO BANANA SMOOTHIE 56
41. SPINACH BLUEBERRY SMOOTHIE 57

42.	SNOWMAN CHRISTMAS SMOOTHIE	57
43.	CLEAN GREEN SHAMROCK SHAKE	57
44.	PUMPKIN SMOOTHIE	58
45.	PROTEIN BALLS WITH PEANUT BUTTER AND CHOCOLATE CHIPS	58
46.	COOKIE DOUGH BALLS	58
47.	GLUTEN-FREE PUMPKIN PIE BARS	59
48.	HEALTHY VEGAN BROWNIES	59
49.	CHOCOLATE CHIA PUDDING	60
50.	GREEN SMOOTHIE RECIPE	60
51.	KEY LIME MOUSSE	61
52.	FUDGY SWEET POTATO BROWNIES	61
53.	BREAKFAST SMOOTHIE	62
54.	POTATO LEEK SOUP	62
55.	TOMATO PASTA BAKE WITH GARLICKY CRUMB TOPPING	63
56.	CREAMY CAULIFLOWER HORSERADISH SOUP	64
57.	CARROT SOUP	64
58.	STRAWBERRY OVERNIGHT OATS	65
59.	GINGER PEACH SMOOTHIE	65
60.	STRAWBERRY BANANA PEANUT BUTTER SMOOTHIE	65
61.	GRANOLA	66
62.	PERSIMMON SMOOTHIE	66
63.	CRANBERRY SMOOTHIE	67
64.	KALE APPLE SMOOTHIE	67
65.	GLOWING SKIN SMOOTHIE	67
66.	CRANBERRY SAUCE	68
67.	CHOCOLATE TAHINI PUMPKIN SMOOTHIE	69
68.	CARAMEL SAUCE	69
69.	LEMON CHEESECAKE SMOOTHIE	69
70.	DOUBLE CHOCOLATE SCONES	70

CHAPTER 6: LUNCH (CLEAR FLUIDS) 72

71.	TROPICAL SMOOTHIE (PINEAPPLE, PAPAYA, COCONUT, LIME SMOOTHIE)	72
72.	CHICKEN BROTH	72
73.	CHICKEN DETOX SOUP	73
74.	BANANA OAT SHAKE	73
75.	BANANA-APPLE SMOOTHIE	74
76.	BERRYLICIOUS SMOOTHIE	74
77.	BUTTERMILK HERB RANCH DRESSING	74
78.	CITRUS RELISH	75
79.	CHICKPEA PANCAKES RECIPE	75
80.	RED WINE SANGRIA RECIPE	76
81.	SALTY DOG COCKTAIL RECIPE	76
82.	SIMPLE SYRUP	76
83.	ROSE SANGRIA RECIPE	77
84.	CHAMPAGNE HOLIDAY PUNCH RECIPE	77
85.	WHITE SANGRIA	77
86.	RASPBERRY MOJITOS WITH BASIL	78
87.	MARGARITA RECIPE	78
88.	PINK GRAPEFRUIT MARGARITA	79

89.	GRAPEFRUIT BASIL SORBET	79
90.	BRULEED GRAPEFRUIT (PAMPLEMOUSSE BRÛLÉ)	80
91.	FROZEN BEERITAS RECIPE	80
92.	SPICY PINEAPPLE HABANERO MARGARITAS	80
93.	CRANBERRY POMEGRANATE MARGARITA WITH SPICED RIM	81
94.	PEACH MILKSHAKE (COPYCAT CHIK-FIL-A PEACH SHAKE RECIPE!)	81
95.	JUGO VERDE (GREEN JUICE)	82
96.	PERFECT MANHATTAN RECIPE	82
97.	FROZEN COCONUT MOJITO	82
98.	MULLED LEMONADE RECIPE	83
99.	CUCUMBER ROSE APEROL SPRITZ	83
100.	PINK GRAPEFRUIT MARGARITA	83
101.	STRAWBERRY MARGARITA RECIPE	84
102.	LARGE-BATCH GOOMBAY SMASH CARIBBEAN COCKTAILS	84
103.	HEALTHY VEGAN BROWNIES	85
104.	GREEN CHICKEN SOUP	85
105.	GREEN RISOTTO RECIPE	86
106.	RASPBERRY MOJITOS WITH BASIL	86
107.	DRUNKEN MONKEY COCKTAIL	87
108.	NEGRONI RECIPE	87
109.	POG PUNCH HAWAIIAN COCKTAIL	87
110.	MULLED WINE (WASSAIL RECIPE)	88
111.	FRENCH LAVENDER LEMONADE RECIPE	88
112.	FROZEN LEMONADE WITH PINEAPPLE	89
113.	CUCUMBER ROSE APEROL SPRITZ	89
114.	THE BEST MARGARITA RECIPE	89
115.	SPICY PINEAPPLE HABANERO MARGARITAS	90
116.	WHOLEMEAL SODA BREAD	90
117.	STRAWBERRY MARGARITA RECIPE	91
118.	CRANBERRY POMEGRANATE MARGARITA WITH SPICED RIM	91
119.	HABANERO MARGARITAS	92
120.	BAHAMIAN BLASTER PARTY PUNCH RECIPE	92
121.	CHAMPAGNE HOLIDAY PUNCH RECIPE	92
122.	PERFECT MANHATTAN RECIPE	93
123.	CHOCOLATE GUINNESS FLOAT RECIPE	93
124.	BERRY BLAST NIMBU PANI	93
125.	SALMON GRILLED WITH SWEET AND SOUR PINEAPPLE SALSA	94
126.	AHI TUNA BURGERS WITH GRILLED PINEAPPLE	94
127.	LEMONADE FUDGE	95
128.	PINK LEMONADE CUPCAKES	95
129.	SALTY DOG COCKTAIL RECIPE	96
130.	GRAPEFRUIT SPARKLER	96
131.	GRAPEFRUIT BASIL SORBET	97
132.	PINK GRAPEFRUIT MARGARITA	97
1.	BRULEED GRAPEFRUIT (PAMPLEMOUSSE BRÛLÉ)	98
133.	BEST MAI TAI COCKTAIL RECIPE	98
134.	LAVENDER MEYER LEMON TOM COLLINS COCKTAIL	99
135.	BRANDY JAVA ICE	99
136.	LAVENDER MEYER LEMON TOM COLLINS COCKTAIL	99

137.	WINE PUNCH COCKTAILS	100
138.	BLASTER PARTY PUNCH RECIPE	100
139.	SMASH CARIBBEAN COCKTAILS	101
140.	CRANBERRY SMOOTHIE	101
141.	NO-WAIT FROSÉ RECIPE	101
142.	LT. DAN'S BEST BLOODY MARY MIX RECIPE (HOMEMADE!)	102
143.	THAI COCONUT CURRY LENTIL SOUP	102
144.	MINT JULEP (RECIPE)	103
145.	KILLER BEE COCKTAILS	103
146.	SPARKLING PINEAPPLE MINT JUICE	103
147.	SWEET TEA OLD FASHIONED COCKTAIL	104
148.	FROZEN BEERITAS RECIPE	104
149.	DECAF PEPPERMINT TEA	105
150.	SUGAR-FREE ROOT BEER ICE POPS	105
151.	SYRUP (RECIPE)	105

CHAPTER 7: DINNER (CLEAR FLUIDS) 106

152.	SWEET TEA	106
153.	CANDIED ORANGE PEEL RECIPE	106
154.	HOT BUTTERED RUM RECIPE	106
155.	CARAMEL HOT APPLE CIDER RECIPE	107
156.	BONITA APPLE COCKTAIL (APPLE BUTTER RUM COCKTAILS)	107
157.	HOT APPLE CIDER WASSAIL RECIPE	108
158.	MANGO SMOOTHIE	108
159.	AUTHENTIC CHAI TEA RECIPE	108
160.	JUGO VERDE (GREEN JUICE)	109
161.	ASIAN BLOODY MARY COCKTAIL	109
162.	AGUA FRESCA	109
163.	SOUTHERN ORANGEADE RECIPE	110
164.	VODKA GUMMY BEARS POPSICLES	110
165.	BAILEYS IRISH CREAM JELLO SHOTS	110
166.	AFFOGATO BOURBON SHOTS	111
167.	HIBISCUS GINGER ICED TEA AND MARTINI	111
168.	CHOCOLATE BRANDY LATTE	112
169.	TOFFEE CARAMEL LATTE	112

CHAPTER 8: SNACKS (CLEAR FLUIDS) 113

170.	LEMON RICOTTA CAKE (CREPE CAKE RECIPE)	113
171.	SWEET FRIED PLANTAINS	114
172.	MANGO PUDDING (DAIRY FREE!) RECIPE	114
173.	FRENCH CHOCOLATE SILK PIE RECIPE	115
174.	PEANUT BUTTER OATMEAL CHOCOLATE CHIP COOKIES (MONSTER COOKIE RECIPE)	116
175.	BANANA OATMEAL CHOCOLATE CHIP COOKIES (HEALTHY!)	117
176.	LARABAR SNACK BAR	117
177.	KULFI INDIAN ICE CREAM	117
178.	EASY NO-BAKE KEY LIME PIE RECIPE	118
179.	LEMON CHEESECAKE RECIPE (LIMONCELLO CAKE!)	118
180.	FRENCH TOAST	119

181.	PINEAPPLE ORANGE CREAMSICLE	120
182.	EASY PEACH COBBLER RECIPE WITH BISQUICK	120
183.	HEALTHY 5-MINUTE STRAWBERRY PINEAPPLE SHERBET	121
184.	BEST COCONUT MILK ICE CREAM (DAIRY-FREE!)	121
185.	LEMON CRINKLE COOKIES RECIPE	122
186.	THE BEST NO-BAKE CHOCOLATE LASAGNA	123
187.	EASIEST HEALTHY WATERMELON SMOOTHIE RECIPE	123
188.	WATERMELON	124
189.	BEST ORANGE JULIUS	124

CHAPTER 9: BREAKFAST (LOW-RESIDUE) 126

190.	CHICKEN VEGETABLE PASTA SOUP	126
191.	BEET CARROT SOUP	126
192.	BROTH BRAISED ASPARAGUS	126
193.	LEMON CHICKEN RICE SOUP	127
194.	"MIXED BAG" KALE SALAD	127
195.	CHICKEN SAFFRON RICE PILAF	127
196.	VANILLA SOY PUDDING	128
197.	VANILLA PEAR RASPBERRY PANNA COTTA	128
198.	EGG POTATO BITES	129
199.	BROCCOLI RED EGG BITES	129
200.	BREAKFAST SHRIMP EGG WHITE MUFFIN CUPS	130
201.	GARLICKY CHEESY BROCCOLI GRATIN	130
202.	STEAMED BROCCOLI WITH MISO PEANUT BUTTER SAUCE	131
203.	TOMATO POTATO SAUSAGE PESTO FRITTATA RECIPE	131
204.	SKINNY LOADED STUFFED BAKED POTATO SOUP	132
205.	SWEET POTATO CASSEROLE WITH PRALINE TOPPING	132
206.	CREAMY GARLIC MASHED CAULIFLOWER AND POTATOES	133
207.	CAULIFLOWER MASHED POTATOES WITH TRUFFLE OIL	134
208.	HEALTHY BACON EGG POTATO BREAKFAST CASSEROLE	134
209.	LEMON-BLUEBERRY MUFFINS	135
210.	LEMON-RASPBERRY SAUCE	135

CHAPTER 10: LUNCH (LOW-RESIDUE) 136

211.	SOUTHERN SHRUB	136
212.	ROSEMARY LIME KISS	136
213.	RUBY RED PUNCH	136
214.	EGGY DEVILS	137
215.	CARAMEL SAUCED ORANGES	137
216.	PULLED CHICKEN SALAD	138
217.	BEETROOT CARROT SALAD	138
218.	LEMONGRASS BEEF	139
219.	MANGO PRAWN POKE BOWL	139
220.	CITRUS SWORDFISH	139
221.	HONEY-HERB CHICKEN	140
222.	RED ROSEMARY VINEGAR	140
223.	HERB-CRUSTED TILAPIA	140
224.	STIR-FRY VELVETED CHICKEN AND VEGETABLES	141

CHAPTER 11: DINNER (LOW-RESIDUE) 143

225.	BACON & BALSAMIC TOMATOES	143
226.	CHOCOLATE-CHIPOTLE SIRLOIN STEAK	143
227.	CHEESE SAUCE	143
228.	CROCKPOT CREAM CHEESE CHICKEN	144
229.	2 MINUTE FLOURLESS ENGLISH MUFFIN	144
230.	POTATOES RECIPE	144
231.	PEANUT BUTTER AND JELLY PB&J SMOOTHIE	145
232.	CHOCOLATE MASON JAR ICE CREAM	145
233.	DRY RUB RIBS	145
234.	PROSCIUTTO & SPINACH EGG CUPS	146

CHAPTER 12: BREAKFAST (FIBER-RICH) 147

235.	HIGH-FIBRE MUESLI	147
236.	MEXICAN BEAN SOUP WITH GUACAMOLE	147
237.	WHOLEMEAL SODA BREAD	147
238.	SCRAMBLED EGGS	148
239.	STRAWBERRY BREAKFAST CAKE	148
240.	BLUEBERRY PROTEIN SHAKE	149
241.	CHICKPEA SCRAMBLE BREAKFAST BOWL	149
242.	3-INGREDIENT CHOCOLATE CEREAL	150
243.	VEGGIE QUICHE WITH SWEET POTATO CRUST	150
244.	BLUEBERRY ALMOND OATMEAL	151
245.	GRANOLA YOGURT BREAKFAST TRIFLE	151
246.	LIME MINT SMOOTHIE	151

CHAPTER 13: LUNCH (FIBER-RICH) 152

247.	BLACK BEANS AND AVOCADO TOASTS	152
248.	APPLES N' OATS BREAKFAST SMOOTHIE	152
249.	PACKED BURRITO	152
250.	BLOOD ORANGE CHIA PUDDING	153
251.	BLUEBERRY COCONUT SMOOTHIE BOWL	153
252.	NO-BAKE APRICOT OAT PROTEIN BARS	153
253.	SPRINGTIME TOFU SCRAMBLE	154
254.	DATE-SWEETENED BANANA BREAD	154
255.	2 MINUTE FLOURLESS ENGLISH MUFFIN	155
256.	BLUEBERRY CHIA JAM	155
257.	PEANUT BUTTER CHIA OVERNIGHT OATS	156
258.	PUMPKIN PIE CHIA PUDDING	156
259.	PUMPKIN PIE BUTTER	157
260.	SPICED PUMPKIN GRANOLA	157
261.	COCONUT ALMOND PROTEIN BARS	158
262.	GRAIN-FREE GRANOLA CLUSTERS	158
263.	TOASTED COCONUT AND BERRY GRAIN	159
264.	BERRY SOFT SERVE & VANILLA CHIA PUDDING PARFAIT	160
265.	RAW GRANOLA CLUSTERS, COCONUT WHIPPED CREAM, AND DREAMY BERRY PARFAIT	160
266.	CREAMY RASPBERRY, COCONUT & CHIA SHAKE	161
267.	RAW CHERRY-APPLE PIE	161
268.	STRAWBERRY-WATERMELON REFRESHER JUICE	162

269.	BLUEBERRY BIRCHER POTS	162
270.	JACKET POTATOES WITH HOME-BAKED BEANS	162
271.	PEA & BROAD BEAN SHAKSHUKA	163
272.	LENTIL FRITTERS	163
273.	SUMMER PISTOU	164
274.	WINTER VEGETABLE & LENTIL SOUP	164
275.	BAKED SWEET POTATOES & BEANS	165

DINNER (FIBER-RICH) 166

276.	EASY PEA & SPINACH CARBONARA	166
277.	SAUTÉED BROCCOLI WITH PEANUT SAUCE	166
278.	SPINACH-STRAWBERRY SALAD WITH FETA &	167
279.	SALMON-STUFFED AVOCADOS	167
280.	BEEFLESS TACOS	167
281.	AVOCADO PESTO	168
282.	MEDITERRANEAN CHICKPEA QUINOA BOWL	168
283.	PROSCIUTTO PIZZA WITH ARUGULA	169
284.	TEX-MEX PASTA SALAD	169
285.	BARBECUE PULLED JACKFRUIT SANDWICHES	170
286.	CHERRY TOMATO & GARLIC PASTA	170

CHAPTER 14: SNACKS (FIBER-RICH) 172

287.	ZUCCHINI-CHICKPEA VEGGIE BURGERS WITH TAHINI-RANCH SAUCE	172
288.	CHICKPEA BURGERS & TAHINI SAUCE	172
289.	FALAFEL BURGERS	173
290.	MUSHROOM-QUINOA VEGGIE BURGERS WITH SPECIAL SAUCE	174
291.	CILANTRO BEAN BURGERS WITH CREAMY AVOCADO-LIME SLAW	174
292.	ROSEMARY ALMOND FLOUR PUMPKIN BREAD	175
293.	ORANGE ZUCCHINI BREAD	176
294.	NUT AND BREAD	177
295.	PUMPKIN STUFFED DOUGH BALLS	177
296.	HOMEMADE GRAHAM CRACKERS	178
297.	APPLE AND OAT PANCAKES	179
298.	BLACKBERRY QUINOA BREAKFAST BOWL	179
299.	PROTEIN MUFFINS (5 Ingredients:!)	180

YOUR 30-DAY MEAL PLAN 181
CONCLUSION 186
Recipe Index 188

Printed in Great Britain
by Amazon